SHORT STAY MANAGEMENT OF HEART FAILURE

W. Frank Peacock, IV, MD, FACEP

Vice Chief, Department of Emergency Medicine
Medical Director, Event Medicine
The Cleveland Clinic
Cleveland, Ohio

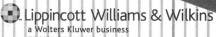

Lippincott Williams & Wilkins
a Wolters Kluwer business
Philadelphia · Baltimore · New York · London
Buenos Aires · Hong Kong · Sydney · Tokyo

Acquisitions Editor: Fran DeStefano
Managing Editor: Nicole Dernoski
Production Manager: Bridgett Dougherty
Manufacturing Manager: Kathleen Brown
Marketing Manager: Angela Panetta
Design Coordinator: Doug Smock
Production Services: Nesbitt Graphics, Inc.
Printer: RR Donnelley

Library of Congress Cataloging-in-Publication Data

Short stay management of heart failure / [edited by] W. Frank Peacock.
  p. ; cm.
  Includes bibliographical references and index.
  ISBN 0-7817-6645-1
  1. Heart failure--Handbooks, manuals, etc.   I. Peacock, W. Frank.
  [DNLM: 1. Heart Failure, Congestive--drug therapy--Handbooks.
  2. Emergency Service, Hospital--organization & administration--Hand-
  books. 3. Observation--Handbooks.   WG 39 S559 2006]
RC685.C53S46 2006
616.1'29--dc22

                        2006004703

Care has been taken to confirm the accuracy of the information presented and to describe generally accepted practices. However, the authors, editors, and publisher are not responsible for errors or omissions or for any consequences from application of the information in this book and make no warranty, expressed or implied, with respect to the currency, completeness, or accuracy of the contents of the publication. Application of this information in a particular situation remains the professional responsibility of the practitioner.

The authors, editors, and publisher have exerted every effort to ensure that drug selection and dosage set forth in this text are in accordance with current recommendations and practice at the time of publication. However, in view of ongoing research, changes in government regulations, and the constant flow of information relating to drug therapy and drug reactions, the reader is urged to check the package insert for each drug for any change in indications and dosage and for added warnings and precautions. This is particularly important when the recommended agent is a new or infrequently employed drug.

Some drugs and medical devices presented in this publication have Food and Drug Administration (FDA) clearance for limited use in restricted research settings. It is the responsibility of the health care provider to ascertain the FDA status of each drug or device planned for use in their clinical practice.

To purchase additional copies of this book, call our customer service department at (800) 638 -3030 or fax orders to (301) 223-2320. International customers should call (301) 223-2300.

Visit Lippincott Williams & Wilkins on the Internet: at LWW.com. Lippincott Williams & Wilkins customer service representatives are available from 8:30 am to 6pm, EST.

10 9 8 7 6 5 4 3 2 1

CONTRIBUTORS

Nancy M. Albert, PhD, CCNS, CCRN, CNA

Adjunct Associate Professor, Frances Payne Bolton School of Nursing, Case Western Reserve University; Director of Nursing Research and Innovation, The Cleveland Clinic, Cleveland, Ohio

Douglas S. Ander, MD

Associate Professor and Director of Undergraduate Education, Department of Emergency Medicine, Emory University School of Medicine, Atlanta, Georgia

Arti N. Bhavsar, PharmD

Assistant Director, Clinical Services, Department of Pharmacy, Florida Hospital, Orlando, Florida

Sean P. Collins, MD, MSc

Assistant Professor, Department of Emergency Medicine, University of Cincinnati, Cincinnati, Ohio

Ginger A. Conway, MSN, RN, CNP

Field Service Instructor, Department of Internal Medicine, Division of Cardiology, University of Cincinnati, Cincinnati, Ohio

Deborah B. Diercks, MD, FACEP

Associate Professor of Emergency Medicine, University of California, Davis Medical Center, Sacramento, California

Harischandra B. Karunaratne, MD

Director of Coronary Care Unit and Co Director of Cardiovascular Research, Department of Cardiology, Florida Hospital, Orlando, Florida

J. Douglas Kirk, MD, FACEP

Associate Professor of Emergency Medicine, Vice Chair for Clinical Operations, Medical Director, Chest Pain Evaluation Unit, Department of Emergency Medicine, University of California, Davis, Medical Center, Sacramento, California

Vincent N. Mosesso Jr., MD

Associate Professor of Emergency Medicine, University of Pittsburgh School of Medicine and Medical Director of Prehospital Care, University of Pittsburgh Medical Center, Pittsburgh, Pennsylvania

W. Frank Peacock, IV, MD, FACEP

Vice Chief, Emergency Medicine, Medical Director, Event Medicine, The Cleveland Clinic, Cleveland, Ohio

Majid J. Qazi, DO

Cardiology Fellow, Botsford General Hospital, Farmington Hills, Michigan

Nicole Rosenke

Student, Department of Pharmacy, Florida Hospital, Orlando, Florida

Elsie M. Selby MSN, ARNP, CCNS, CCRN

Director, Cardiopulmonary Services/Sleep Disorder Center, Ephraim McDowell Regional Medical Center, Danville, Kentucky

Sandra Sieck, RN, MBA

President and CEO, Sieck HealthCare Consulting, Mobile, Alabama

Robert J. Stomel, DO

Assistant Clinical Profesor, Department of Internal Medicine, Michigan State University, East Lansing, Michigan; Chief of Cardiology, Department of Cardiology/Internal Medicine, Botsford General Hospital, Farmington Hills, Michigan

Robin J. Trupp, MSN, APRN, BC, CCRN

President, Comprehensive CV Consulting LLC, PhD Student, College of Nursing, The Ohio State University, Columbus, Ohio

Marvin A. Wayne, MD, FACEP

Associate Clinical Professor, School of Medicine, University of Washington, Seattle, Washington; Senior Attending Physician, Department of Emergency Medicine, St. Joseph Hospital, Bellingham, Washington

TABLE OF CONTENTS

1

HEART FAILURE IN THE OBSERVATION UNIT

W. F. Peacock

WHY HEART FAILURE?

Plain and simple, heart failure is the number one disease in our country. This is a poorly recognized fact that results from the confluence of society's excesses with the medical community's success in staving off the inevitable consequences of sedentary overconsumption and self-indulgence. Because we live at a time and in a place where myocardial infarction is not a uniformly fatal event, where obesity exists in epidemic proportions, where the coronary artery stent and coronary artery bypass graft (CABG) are part of the routine layperson's coffee table vernacular, and where hypertensive and diabetic individuals routinely live for scores of years after their diagnosis, we have created an entire subpopulation of Americans who survive with serious compromise to their cardiovascular function.

As recently as 30 years ago, these patients simply died of complications from their diseases. Today they commonly survive, only to reenter the medical establishment in later years with the development of heart failure. Thus, heart failure has become the disease of the 21st century. It is also the chronic ailment that steals the quality of life from the golden years of America's fastest growing demographic segment: the elderly. No other single disease causes more hospitalizations, and few other pathologies can as effectively maim and suffocate its victims, as heart failure is routinely manifested.

Unfortunately, in its early stages, heart failure is relatively asymptomatic and passes unnoticed until the patient presents with symptoms of progressive shortness of breath. Although the patient may give a history of a relatively new onset of dysfunction, in reality the underlying syndrome has been present chronically, sometimes for years. It is the symptom of suffocation that drives heart failure patients to the emergency department. As has been shown in data from the ADHERE registry, more than 90% of heart failure patients present acutely with shortness of breath. It is ultimately dyspnea that results in their hospitalization and it is breathlessness that is the limiting parameter preventing their discharge home. Consequently, the relief of shortness of breath becomes the driving event determining both the length of hospitalization required and the quality of life in the heart failure patient.

Heart failure has been termed the "merry-go-round" disease. This is because of the well-known cycle of worsening symptoms, hospital admission, discharge home, followed by worsening symptoms and repeat of the same cycle. If only it were so. The unfortunate reality is that the long-term course of heart failure more resembles a roller coaster than a merry-go-round. On a merry-go-round, the cycle is repeated and the patient returns to where he or she started. However, on a roller coaster, the highest level of function is the first day, and it is all downhill from there. In heart failure, the patient is initially functional, worsens, and is hospitalized and is discharged, usually not in as good a condition as when first stricken, only to repeat this cycle. Therefore, what seems like a repeating cycle is actually a downward spiral ending inevitably, usually within 5 years, with the patient's death.

This roller coaster ride is not good for the patient. Constant repeat visits and the expensive polypharmacy that defines contemporary heart failure management serve to steal quality of life and robs the patient of his or her life savings. It is not just the patient who is financially burdened. Heart failure costs the medical establishment huge sums of money. The Center for Medicare and Medicaid Studies spends more on heart failure care than on any other single disease.

Solutions to this problem, both from the patient's point of view and from the perspective of the health care provider, are sorely needed. Business as usual has been a dismal failure for the treatment of heart failure. The number of heart failure hospitalizations has dramatically risen over the last 30 years and will surpass 1 million in 2005. When we consider that the most common heart failure patient in the ADHERE registry is a 75-year-old white woman, the future is daunting. All demographic projections of an aging United States suggest that the number of people stricken with heart failure can only markedly increase.

New and creative solutions must be implemented. This book represents the first of its kind to focus on acute decompensated heart failure treatment without conventional hospitalization. Our goals are to improve the patient's quality of life by avoiding hospitalizations and to do so in a financially effective manner.

HAVING TO GO FIRST IS HARDER THAN IT LOOKS

I have often wondered when humans were first faced with the necessity of digging a hole, how did they come to decide to make a shovel? It is a pretty rudimentary object, a relatively small piece of metal plate with a curved shape, a point at one end, and a place where the handle goes. It was most certainly not invented by a rocket scientist. But what if you had never seen one? What if metal had not even been invented? Would the shovel be the first tool you would spend your time making? After all, remember, you just needed a hole. So it is likely that the first shovel probably looked more like a stick. And that is the conundrum of going first. The final solution to any given problem will likely not resemble the answer to the challenge that was the original objective, and so it is with heart failure. This is the first book to tackle the problem of digging out of the hole that we currently know as heart failure. We hope it will not be the last. We hope, too, that this represents the first in a long chain of refinements toward the goal of meeting the challenge of the number one disease in America.

CLARIFICATION OF TERMS

Throughout this manuscript little attempt has been made to standardize terms. This represents the current state of the literature, as much as the billing structure that drives the medical establishment. Whether the unit is called an emergency department observation unit, a short stay unit, or a rapid diagnostic and treatment unit is unimportant. Whether it is managed by emergency physicians, internists, cardiologists, or nurse practitioners is superfluous. Finally, whether it is in a specialized location with dedicated beds and equipment or a virtual unit with no defined geography, the desired outcome remains the same. The common goal, and the objective of this book, is that all heart failure patients receive early diagnosis and effective treatment that allows a rapid discharge that does not require a revisit within 30 days.

Thus, in reality, standardization of terms is irrelevant. The intent of this book is to outline strategies for the early diagnosis and treatment of the acutely decompensated heart failure patient in a "short stay unit." What a "short stay unit" is has intentionally been left vague. The geography of where the care occurs or the medical background of the practitioners has little relevance. What is important is a common dedication to improving outcomes for patients presenting with acutely decompensated heart failure.

ON THE SHOULDERS OF GIANTS

No introduction to this book could possibly be complete without the appropriate thanks to those who have made this book possible. For this, we stand on the shoulders of two giants. It was in Michigan, in the last decade of the 20th century when Dr. Raymond Bahr, a forward-thinking cardiologist, brought to fruition his idea of a new society dedicated to the care of the chest pain patient. Many years later, this ultimately came to be what we now know as the Society for Chest Pain. Interestingly, like the man who just needed to dig a hole, there was no way for Ray to know that, many years later, the society he formed in the basement of a Detroit hotel would become the standard bearer for heart failure and serve to spawn an entirely different perspective of care for entire groups of patients. Much thanks must go to Ray for his ability to think outside the box.

Second, due thanks must be given to Lou Graff who, in the same decade, published the first-ever book on rapid diagnosis and treatment units. Titled *Observation Medicine,* this book became the standard bearer and served as the "how to" manual for many subsequent hospitals to organize their observation units. Without the confluence of chest pain units, supported and advanced by Ray Bahr, and the concept of observation medicine, defined and promoted by Lou Graff, the necessary pieces to care for heart failure patients in a short stay unit would not exist today.

It is our hope that this book will perform in a manner similar to its predecessors, in the fashion of assisting practitioners in the search for new ways to improve outcomes for their patients' quality of life and their hospital partners.

2

THE OUT-OF-HOSPITAL MANAGEMENT OF ACUTE HEART FAILURE

Marvin A. Wayne and Vincent N. Mosesso, Jr.

INTRODUCTION

Acute heart failure (AHF) is one of only two cardiovascular diseases with an increasing prevalence; the other is atrial fibrillation. Five million Americans have the disease, and more than 500,000 are newly diagnosed each year. AHF is a major disease of our aging population[1] because most hospitalizations for AHF are of patients older than 65 years.[2] Heart failure (HF) results in more than 2 million hospitalizations annually and accounts for about 3% of the national health care budget.[1] Further, it is Medicare's largest single disease expenditure. Approximately 300,000 deaths are annually related to HF.[3]

Heart failure, and its acute presentation, AHF, is a complex disease that includes at least four clinical syndromes: exacerbation of chronic HF, hypertensive crisis, acute pulmonary edema (APE), and cardiogenic shock.[4] Of these four syndromes, APE and cardiogenic shock are the two most serious. Although the major clinical manifestations in both are a combination of decreased peripheral perfusion and pulmonary congestion, they differ in pathophysiology and hemodynamic changes. Accordingly, these syndromes require different therapeutic approaches.

APE, the most common clinical manifestation of AHF,[5] is a life-threatening respiratory emergency usually occurring in the out-of-hospital setting. The overall prehospital mortality rate for APE in a retrospective Italian study has been reported to be 8%.[6] Although similar data for the United States are not readily available, a favorable outcome for AHF is dependent on rapid assessment and treatment initiated in the out-of-hospital setting.

PATHOGENESIS OF APE

APE can be of a cardiogenic or noncardiogenic etiology. In the former, pulmonary edema results from increased microvascular hydrostatic pressure, whereas in the latter edema arises from increased pulmonary capillary

TABLE 2-1 Precipitating Causes of Acute Cardiogenic Pulmonary Edema (APE)

Cause	Incidence (%)
Worsening heart failure	26
Coronary insufficiency	21
Subendocardial infarction	16
Transmural infarction	10
Acute dysrhythmia	9
Medication noncompliance	7
Dietary indiscretion	3
Valvular insufficiency	3
Other	5

From Marx J, Hockberger R, Walls R. *Rosen's emergency medicine: concepts and clinical practice,* 5th ed. Saint Louis: Mosby, 2002, with permission.

permeability. The end result is identical in both cases: an excessive accumulation of extravascular lung fluid.[7] The primary cause of cardiogenic APE is cardiac dysfunction (Table 2-1). Noncardiogenic APE may be caused by several diverse events or diseases, which include systemic or pulmonary infection, trauma, septic shock, toxic inhalation, or aspiration of gastric contents.[8] Because both types of APE have the same clinical manifestations—dyspnea, diaphoresis, decreased lung compliance, anxiety, and increased shunt fraction—distinguishing between the two can be extremely difficult.[7]

APE is often difficult to distinguish clinically from an exacerbation of chronic obstructive pulmonary disease (COPD) or other acute pulmonary disorders. The misdiagnosis of AHF in the out-of-hospital setting has been documented to be 23% in one study[9] and as high as 32% in another.[10] The need for the correct identification of precipitating events, and the rapid initiation of appropriate treatment, is critical to achieve a positive outcome. Inappropriate therapy, as a result of misdiagnosis, may result in harm to the patient. Hoffman and Reynolds[9] reported that adverse effects were more common in misdiagnosed patients. Untoward effects included (a) respiratory depression in patients receiving morphine, (b) hypotension and bradycardia in patients receiving both morphine and nitroglycerin, and (c) arrhythmia associated with hypokalemia in patients receiving furosemide.

Initiating events or conditions, including myocardial ischemia, hypertensive crisis, fluid excess, medication noncompliance, diet, and overexertion, may trigger AHF. Each may set in motion a vicious cycle of events that results in cardiogenic APE. The key components of this cycle, outlined in Figure 2-1, all involve left ventricular (LV) dysfunction.[11] A marked increase in systemic vascular resistance in conjunction with impaired myocardial

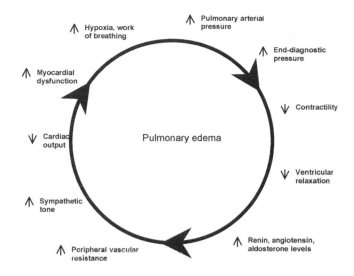

FIGURE 2-1 Processes involved in pulmonary edema. Cycle may begin at any point but once begun is self-perpetuating. (From Sacchetti AD, Harris RH. Acute cardiogenic pulmonary edema. What's the latest in emergency treatment? *Postgrad Med* 1998;103:145–147, with permission.)

contractility, from either systolic or diastolic dysfunction, results in pulmonary edema. This increase in vascular resistance leads to an increase in LV diastolic pressure resulting in increased pulmonary venous pressure. This increases hydrostatic pressure, which then forces fluid to leak out of the pulmonary capillaries into the pulmonary interstitial space and alveoli, producing edema. As edema worsens, so does oxygen diffusion, and thus oxygen saturation drops and further compromises cardiac contractility, creating a positive feedback circuit.[12]

Field Assessment

Assessment begins with a rapid, focused history and physical examination of the patient. This includes patient history, recent illness, prescribed medications, medication compliance, and diet. Together this constitutes an important first step in the field diagnosis of AHF (Table 2–2). Critical elements of the physical examination include accurate determination of vital signs. AHF/APE is often associated with marked elevation in systolic blood pressure. Prehospital providers, even in the absence of peripheral edema, should strongly consider cardiogenic pulmonary edema in patients presenting with acute respiratory distress, hypoxemia, tachypnea, rales or wheezing, and marked hypertension. Such patients often have histories of poorly controlled hypertension and/or prior cardiac disease. Blood pressure of greater than 180/120 mm Hg is common in this setting and is a good sign of reversibility. In these patients, a rapid reduction in blood pressure often produces prompt relief of respiratory distress. Marked

TABLE 2–2 **Diagnosis of Congestive Heart Failure**

Prior history and comorbid states

- Chronic heart failure
- Hypertension
- Ischemic heart disease
- Valvular heart disease
- Anemia
- Dysrhythmias
- Thyroid disease

Current situation

- Medications (prescribed regimen and current compliance, other drug use)
- Symptoms of acute coronary syndromes
- Diet or exercise indiscretions in patients with known heart failure
- Signs of pulmonary edema such as tachypnea, low oxygen saturation, rales, and peripheral edema
- Signs of chronic obstructive pulmonary disease, asthma, or airway obstruction
- Signs of pneumonia or sepsis, such as fever and purulent sputum

Tools

- Pulse oximetry
- End-tidal carbon dioxide trends
- ECG rhythm and 12-lead if does not delay transport

Potential future diagnostic aids

- B-type natriuretic peptide
- Noninvasive cardiac output
- Correlated audio electrocardiography

ECG, electrocardiogram.

hypertension associated with acute respiratory distress and wheezing, particularly in elderly patients without a history of asthma or pulmonary infection, is strongly suggestive of APE. Such a presumptive diagnosis may be supported by the presence of cardiovascular medications and the absence of respiratory medications, such as metered-dose inhalers. Even when these facts are present, out-of-hospital personnel should always consider alternate etiologies such as pulmonary embolism, pneumonia, asthma, and drug overdose before diagnosing patients as having APE. Although rhythm strips and standard 12-lead electrocardiograms (ECGs) are useful in identifying arrhythmia and/or acute coronary syndrome, they are insensitive and nonspecific for diagnosing AHF.[13,14] Furthermore, these ECGs and rhythm strip tracings may be prone to misinterpretation.[15] Recently, a new type of ECG has been developed. This system uses an acoustic sensor at leads V_3 and V_4 to diagnose the presence of S_3 and/or S_4 heart sounds (Audicor Inovice Medical Systems, Portland, OR). The presence of an S_3 in patients older than 45 years is highly specific for the presence of HF and may aid in the diagnosis of AHF.[15,16]

In addition to these diagnostic tests, a number of other diagnostic aids have been developed to improve accuracy in the evaluation and diagnosis of AHF. Although not currently used in the prehospital environment, a rapid bedside assay of blood levels of B-type natriuretic peptide, a neurohormone secreted mainly by the cardiac ventricles in response to volume expansion and pressure overload, is useful in establishing or excluding the diagnosis of AHF in patients with acute dyspnea in the emergency department (ED).[16-21] Application of such testing in the out-of-hospital environment may be a logical extension and further aid in diagnosis. Currently, noninvasive cardiac output (NICO) devices, such as impedance cardiography,[22] have also been suggested as diagnostic tools, but their complexities and cost have to date precluded their out-of-hospital use.

MANAGEMENT OF APE

Fluid accumulation in the lungs associated with APE, until recently, was attributed to excess accumulation of total body fluid. Accordingly, treatment of APE was aimed at removing excess fluid by promoting massive diuresis. However, this explanation did not reconcile with APE cases without an increase in total body water. The current explanation is that APE results from fluid redistribution within the body whereby a part of the intravascular volume is redistributed to the lungs as a consequence of increased intravascular pressure.[12] Primary objectives for the treatment of AHF and associated APE are to reduce pulmonary capillary pressure, to redistribute pulmonary fluid, and to improve forward flow.[11,12] These goals may be achieved by reducing LV preload and afterload, providing ventilatory and inotropic supports, and identifying and treating the underlying etiology of the syndrome (Table 2–3). It should be recognized that these treatment measures are intended for APE patients who are normotensive or

TABLE 2–3 Management of Acute Congestive Heart Failure: Overview

- Identify CHF
- Identify and treat specific etiology when possible
- Provide oxygen and ventilatory support when needed
- Reduce LV preload
- Reduce LV afterload
- Provide inotropic support when needed
- Match receiving facility with needed resources

CHF, congestive heart failure; LV, left ventricular.

hypertensive and not those who are hypotensive. The latter comprises cardiogenic shock arising secondary to severe LV systolic dysfunction; these patients may need inotropic or mechanical cardiac support, and the treatment of these critically ill patients is beyond the scope of this review.

Reduction of LV Preload

The initial effort to reduce the pulmonary congestion in patients presenting with APE should be to reduce the pressure and volume of blood flow to the pulmonary vasculature. This may be accomplished by dilating the venous capacitance system. This will result in decreased blood return to the right ventricle (preload), hence reducing blood flow to the pulmonary vascular bed. The net result is a reduction in LV preload, which then allows the LV output to more closely match inflow from the pulmonary system.[11] Pharmacologic therapy to reduce LV preload includes the use of nitrates primarily and, to a more limited extent, morphine and loop diuretics such as furosemide.

NITRATES. Nitroglycerin and related drugs at low dosages are primarily venodilators effective in decreasing pulmonary artery pressure. Intracellularly, they react with and convert sulfhydryl groups to S-nitrosothiols and nitric oxide. These reactive groups then activate the enzyme guanylate cyclase, which catalyzes the formation of cyclic guanosine monophosphate (cGMP). This nucleotide induces the reentry of calcium back into the sarcoplasmic reticulum of vascular smooth muscle thereby causing its relaxation.[23]

Nitroglycerin is currently the vasodilator agent of choice for the reduction of LV preload in the field. It is fast acting, efficient, and easy to administer.[11,12] Nitroglycerin's effectiveness in reducing mortality in patients with APE in the prehospital setting has been demonstrated by Bertini (1997).[6] In this study, even hypotensive patients (systolic blood pressure <100 mm Hg) were found to respond positively to nitroglycerin. Likewise, Hoffman and Reynolds[9] compared a number of prehospital management protocols for APE and concluded that nitroglycerin was beneficial, whereas morphine and furosemide had no additive effect when combined with nitroglycerin and were occasionally deleterious. The beneficial hypotensive effect of nitroglycerin must be closely monitored so that the reduction in blood pressure does not deleteriously reduce LV preload and the ability to produce adequate cardiac output. Thus, a potential disadvantage of nitroglycerin is that it can lead to excessive hypotension,[8] particularly in patients without adequate preload [e.g., hypovolemia and inferior wall myocardial infarction (MI) with significant right ventricular (RV) involvement].

MORPHINE. Although morphine has been used for decades to treat acute MI, unstable angina, and AHF, few clinical trials have demonstrated its effectiveness in acute congestive heart failure (CHF). Its popularity in treating pulmonary edema arose because of its vasodilatory and antianxiety effects, although morphine's vasodilatory effects are transient and are the result of histamine release.[11] Recently, concerns have been raised over the use of morphine in treating acute CHF in the ED. A retrospective study of the ED management of APE and intensive care unit (ICU) admissions showed that morphine administered in the ED was associated with significant increases in ICU admissions and the need for endotracheal intubations (ETIs) when compared with treatment with sublingual captopril.[24] Additionally, a prospective study of morphine use in prehospital APE treatment showed that the drug was minimally effective as single therapy or in combination with nitrates.[9] Furthermore, the effects of morphine in depressing respiration and the central nervous system may be deleterious in misdiagnosed patients.[9]

FUROSEMIDE. Furosemide has been a mainstay of treatment for APE since the 1960s, although its effectiveness has been examined in only a few studies. Its primary mechanism of action involves the inhibition of sodium reabsorption in the ascending limb of Henle's loop in the renal medulla. This results in an increased excretion of salt and water in urine. The net effect of this action is a lowering of plasma volume, a decrease in LV preload, and a decrease in pulmonary congestion. These effects are beneficial in patients presenting with pulmonary volume overload.[25] In addition to its diuretic effects, furosemide also induces neurohumoral changes. These include both vasodilation (by promoting renal prostaglandin E_2 and atrial natriuretic peptide secretion) and vasoconstricting effects.[26] The latter, via the feedback loop, can result in peripheral elevation of mean arterial pressure, LV pressure, heart rate, and systemic vascular resistance through enhancement of the renin-angiotensin system (RAS). Stroke volume index and pulmonary capillary wedge pressure initially decrease but subsequently increase after the RAS enhancement (usually within 15 minutes). The latter effects are not beneficial in the treatment of AHF particularly in the absence of volume overload.[11,12] Furthermore, misdiagnosis of AHF and subsequent inducement of inappropriate diuresis can lead to increased morbidity and mortality in patients with other conditions such as pneumonia, sepsis, or COPD.[9,25]

COMBINED DRUG THERAPIES WITH NITROGLYCERIN, FUROSEMIDE, AND MORPHINE. Nitrates are frequently combined with loop diuretics in treating pulmonary edema. A complex, randomized, prospective clinical study from Israel investigated the efficacy and safety of these drugs in treating patients presenting with severe pulmonary edema in the prehospital setting.[27] This study concluded that intravenous (IV) nitrates administered as repeated high-dose boluses (3 mg every 5 minutes) after a low dose (40 mg) of furosemide was associated with lower ETI and MI rates than the administration of low-dose nitrates (1 mg per hour, increased by 1 mg per hour every 10 minutes) and high-dose furosemide (80 mg every 15 minutes). A prospective observational study on the use of sublingual nitroglycerin in the prehospital setting in cases of presumed MI or CHF analyzed treatment-related adverse events in 300 patients. Only four patients experienced adverse events, most of which were bradycardic-hypotensive reactions, and all recovered subsequently.[28]

A retrospective case review evaluated outcomes of 57 patients presumed to have prehospital APE who were treated in the field with combinations of nitroglycerin, furosemide, and/or morphine.[9] Although only a small study, any combination treatment including nitroglycerin was associated with both subjective and objective (respiratory and heart rates, blood pressure, respiratory distress, mental status) improvement. Combination treatment with furosemide and morphine without nitroglycerin, on the other hand, resulted in a substantial number of patients not responding to treatment and some actually deteriorating. Ultimately, 23 of 57 (47%) patients in this study were found not to have pulmonary edema.

A larger retrospective case series evaluated outcomes in 493 patients receiving prehospital nitroglycerin, furosemide, and/or morphine versus no treatment for CHF. Mortality was significantly reduced in the more critical patients receiving any prehospital drug treatment compared with no treatment (5% vs. 33%, $p < 0.01$) as well as in the entire treated patient population (6.7% vs. 15.4%, $p < 0.01$).[29]

Reduction of LV Afterload

A variety of pharmacologic agents, including nitroglycerin at higher doses, angiotensin-converting enzyme (ACE) inhibitors, nitroprusside, dobutamine, and dopamine, may be useful in the reduction of LV afterload.

NITRATES AT HIGHER DOSES. High-dose nitrates can reduce both preload and afterload and potentially increase cardiac output.[30] Because many CHF patients present with very elevated arterial and venous pressures, frequent doses of nitrates may be required to control blood pressure and afterload. Some patients develop tolerance to nitroglycerin, but this is not of concern in the prehospital environment. Another concern with high-dose nitrates is that certain patients are very sensitive to even normal doses and may experience marked hypotension. These are typically patients with tenuous preload status (e.g., preexisting hypovolemia or significant RV infarction in the setting of inferior wall MI). It is therefore critical to monitor blood pressure during high-dose nitrate therapy.

ACE INHIBITORS. ACE inhibitors play a primary role in chronic CHF therapy and have multiple therapeutic advantages for treating APE. These include reducing both preload and afterload, increasing splanchnic flow, decreasing LV diastolic dysfunction, reducing sodium retention, and reducing sympathetic stimulation. Captopril (Capoten) is an ACE inhibitor that has been studied in the prehospital setting.[11] When a standard tablet is administered sublingually, it rapidly dissolves and has an onset of action of less than 10 minutes. Clinical effects are seen within 15 minutes, with peak effects within 30 minutes.[31,32] A retrospective study of 181 patients with APE treated in the ED examined the relationship between pharmacologic trcatments and rates of ICU admissions.[24] Patients in this study were treated with captopril (26%), nitroglycerin (81%), morphine (49%), and/or loop diuretics (73%). Patients receiving captopril had decreased rates of ICU admissions and ETIs as well as shorter ICU stays. A prospective, placebo-controlled, randomized study evaluated the addition of sublingual captopril to the standard treatment regimen (oxygen, nitrates, morphine, and furosemide) in patients brought to the ED with APE.[32] Using a clinical APE distress score for assessment, the addition of captopril was found to significantly reduce distress scores over the first 40 minutes compared with placebo. This study indicated that certain features of ACE inhibitors make them attractive for field use, including ease of sublingual administration, fast onset of action, and low cost.[11,31,33] However, captopril use may be associated with potential concerns,[34] which include occasional hypotension and a variable duration of effect in comparison to nitrates.

In addition to the sublingual route, ACE inhibitors may also be administered intravenously. Enalaprilat maleate (Vasotec IV) is the only IV ACE inhibitor currently available in the United States,[33] and its efficacy and safety in the treatment of pulmonary edema and CHF have been demonstrated in two small randomized trials.[35,36]

NITROPRUSSIDE. APE patients presenting with severe hypertension and those refractory to nitrate and ACE inhibitor treatments may be candidates for treatment with nitroprusside sodium.[25] However, the need to continuously monitor blood pressure, with a carefully titrated continuous infusion, and the requirement of glass containers shielded from light preclude its utility in the field environment.[24]

Ventilatory Support

Patients with acute CHF may be treated with a spectrum of ventilatory support modalities based on the patient's clinical condition and comorbid factors. Initial treatment includes oxygen therapy to maintain oxygen saturation of at least 92% to 93% and the use of inhaled bronchodilators when bronchospasm is evident.[25] True bronchospasm may be triggered by interstitial edema, especially in patients with underlying reactive airway disease. A new single isomer β_2 agonist for inhalation, levalbuterol HCl (Xopenex, Sepracor Pharmaceutical, Marlborough, MA), may cause less tachycardia than racemic albuterol, of particular concern in patients with HF or cardiac ischemia.

In severe respiratory failure (ineffective respiratory effort, hypoxemia, hypercarbia), assisted ventilation is needed. Traditionally this has been accomplished in tandem with ETI. However, ETI is a challenge to accomplish effectively in noncomatose, nonparalyzed patients with the limited resources and personnel usually available in the field setting. Further, ETI is associated with various infectious (e.g., nosocomial pneumonia, sinusitis) and noninfectious (e.g., barotrauma; oral, nasal, or laryngeal trauma; respiratory muscle weakness; prolonged weaning) complications.[37-40] To avoid these complications and lengthy ICU stays, noninvasive ventilatory support is being increasingly used. ETI remains necessary when altered mental status requires airway protection or when other patient characteristics prevent the successful application of noninvasive positive pressure ventilation (NIPPV).

NONINVASIVE POSITIVE PRESSURE VENTILATION. Noninvasive positive pressure ventilation (NIPPV), traditionally used for COPD and asthma,[41-45] is now considered an effective adjunct treatment of AHF/APE.[46-50] The therapeutic effect of noninvasive pressure support lies in its ability to increase intra-alveolar pressure. This shifts the flow of fluid back into the pulmonary capillaries and thereby reduces pulmonary congestion. NIPPV decreases the work of breathing and thereby decreases myocardial demand. Two different methods of providing NIPPV are used: continuous positive airway pressure (CPAP), which provides a constant level of positive pressure applied throughout inspiration and exhalation, and bilevel positive airway pressure (BiPAP), which allows provision of higher pressure during inspiration than expiration.[51]

Only a few prehospital studies involving CPAP have been conducted. A Swedish study compared outcomes after treatment for AHF during two time periods: one period of standard therapy consisting of nitroglycerin, furosemide, or both (first period) and one period of intensified treatment with nitroglycerin, furosemide, and CPAP (second period).[5] The use of drug therapy and CPAP in patients increased dramatically from the first period to the second period: nitroglycerin from 4% to 68%, furosemide from 13% to 84%, and CPAP from 4% to 91%. Although a greater percentage of patients in the second group had fulminant pulmonary edema (FPE) on ambulance arrival (60% vs. 78%, $p < 0.001$), at admission to the hospital there was a significant reduction in the percentage with FPE during the second period (93% vs. 76.1%, $p < 0.001$). There was also a significantly lower mean level of serum creatine kinase MB in patients in the second group, implying less myocardial damage. Although there was an improvement in symptoms during transport and less myocardial damage, mortality remained high with no significant difference between treatment groups.

A small prospective case-series analysis on the prehospital use of CPAP by trained paramedics in 19 patients with cardiogenic pulmonary edema showed that none of the patients required field intubation and that hemoglobin oxygen saturation increased from a mean of 83.3% to 95.4% after CPAP administration via a face mask.[10] Two patients intolerant of CPAP required ETI on ED arrival and an additional five patients required ETI within 24 hours. There were no adverse events related to CPAP therapy. These results demonstrate that field use of CPAP is feasible but that certain obstacles need to be overcome. In particular, the authors noted that the paramedic's lack of experience with this therapy led to problems with achieving good mask fit and titrating pressure levels.

BiPAP has been investigated as an alternative to CPAP in a number of conditions but has shown a significant advantage over CPAP only in patients whose respiratory failure is due to COPD exacerbation.[52] A number of individual studies reported some success with BiPAP[53,54] and some problems, including increased rates of MI,[55,56] associated with its use in treating acute CHF.

In an out-of-hospital study of patients with presumed CHF, emergency medical services (EMS) personnel considered the use of BiPAP to be safe and judged this method to improve dyspnea and respiratory distress in their patients.[57] Although oxygen saturation was significantly greater for the BiPAP plus conventional treatment group, compared with the conventional treatment group, treatment times, length of hospital stay, intubation rate, and death rates were not significantly different between the groups.

Of the two types of noninvasive ventilatory support, there is good supporting evidence for the effectiveness of CPAP. New technology appears to make field implementation of CPAP simpler and more efficacious and overcomes some of the earlier concerns about its use. Greater experience of field providers should also lead to better outcomes because this therapy is not only patient dependent but operator dependent as well. In the case of BiPAP, the risk-benefit ratio is conflicting in the literature. In addition, the existing technology for BiPAP is suboptimal for out-of-hospital use. Further field trials investigating the implementation of these modalities and testing technologic refinements are needed.

SUMMARY

This review focuses on the importance of understanding that the pathogenesis of APE is related to intravascular fluid redistribution rather than to primary volume overload (Figure 2–1). Management of suspected APE begins with correct assessment and management of underlying causes of elevated ventricular filling pressures and continues with improving oxygenation with the application of ventilatory support, reduction of LV preload and afterload with nitroglycerin and inotropic support when necessary. Care must be taken with drugs such as furosemide and morphine because patient outcomes can be adversely affected when administered for conditions mimicking APE. EMS personnel must assiduously seek hallmarks of acute CHF as opposed to other medical conditions associated with acute dyspnea. Sophisticated, rapid tools such as quantitative B-type natriuretic peptide (BNP) assays and noninvasive hemodynamic devices may one day provide greater diagnostic accuracy in the field. A guide based on clinical evidence for treating prehospital patients suffering from acute CHF is suggested (Table 2–4).

Nitrates are recommended as first-line therapy for APE in the field with symptom resolution as the primary treatment goal. Nitrates provide both subjective and objective improvement (with high-dose, repeat sublingual or spray administration). Blood pressure is an important gauge of

TABLE 2-4 Classification for Treatment

Class	Characteristics	Treatment	Comments
I Asymptomatic	Dyspnea on exertion but not currently at rest	Provide high flow supplemental O_2 Consider intravenous access	Maintain SaO_2 >93% Saline lock
II Mild symptoms	Mild dyspnea even at rest and despite O_2 treatment Able to speak full sentences If SBP >110 mm Hg	Low-dose nitroglycerin (0.4 mg every 4–5 min) Definite IV access Monitor ECG Chew aspirin Bronchodilator	If no contraindication to nitrates (e.g., sildenafil within 24 hours) and if SBP >110 mm Hg — 12 lead when available If suspect coronary ischemia If wheezing
III Moderate symptoms	Moderate dyspnea (SaO_2 < 95% on O_2) SBP >110 mm Hg Unable to speak full sentences Normal mental status	High-dose SL nitroglycerin Bronchodilator Consider furosemide	If SBP >110 mm Hg If wheezing (use nebulizer if MDI cannot be used) If peripheral edema
IV Severe symptoms	Severe dyspnea-respiratory failure: hypoxia, altered sensorium, diaphoresis, and one-word sentences	High-dose SL nitroglycerin (0.8–2 mg every 3–5 min) Bronchodilators-nebulizers Consider morphine (2–4 mg) Furosemide Consider ETI or NIPPV	Watch carefully for hypotension (use only if SBP >110 mm Hg) Watch for respiratory depression For agitation If peripheral edema If time and patient tolerance permits

ECG, electrocardiogram; ETI, endotracheal intubation; IV, intravenous; MDI, metered-dose inhaler; NIPPV, noninvasive positive pressure ventilation; SaO_2, arterial oxygen saturation; SBP, systolic blood pressure; SL, sublingual.

Treatment at each level should consider the lowest dose where applicable.

effective nitrate dosing. Endpoints should be primarily guided by the patient's level of dyspnea and oxygen saturation and avoidance of hypotension. In patients with systolic blood pressures less than 90 to 100 mm Hg, nitroglycerin should not be routinely administered.

The use of loop diuretics such as furosemide requires careful consideration. Although furosemide is beneficial in transiently decreasing the pulmonary capillary wedge pressure, it can also increase the systemic vascular resistance. The primary concern involves the increased morbidity and mortality associated with prehospital administration of diuretics in conditions that mimic APE and in patients with APE who do not have an excess of total body water. This may occur in patients with new onset HF, such as in association with an acute MI. The use of diuretics in combination with nitrates has also been proved to have no early clinical benefit. In the absence of peripheral edema or other evidence of excess total body water (such as documented acute weight gain), routine diuretic administration should be avoided.

Evidence for the use of ACE inhibitors is not currently sufficient to recommend their use in the prehospital care of APE. Although they have an essential role in chronic HF, the lack of supporting data and potential disadvantages including hypotension, adverse interaction with aspirin, decrease in glomerular filtration rate, and longer duration of action preclude endorsing their use in APE at this time.

Bronchodilator use is appropriate when wheezing is the result of bronchospasm but should not preclude delivery of other specific therapy for CHF, such as nitroglycerin or CPAP. It is not clear whether CPAP or BiPAP provides a consistent outcome advantage. Initial field studies have been promising, but issues such as the need for specialized training in mask adjustment and pressure titration, high-volume oxygen consumption requirement for operation, or suboptimal portability due to the need for an electrical power source present logistical obstacles. New technology may make the field administration of CPAP simpler and more efficacious.

CONCLUSION

APE is a common and often life-threatening condition encountered by prehospital emergency medical personnel. Patients with this condition must receive rapid, accurate assessment and aggressive treatment. High-dose nitrates represent the out-of-hospital treatment of choice, whereas diuretics and morphine should be reserved for select patient groups. More data are needed on the efficacy and safety of ACE inhibitors to justify their use in the field. CPAP has been shown to be effective, but more experience and refinement of delivery systems for the prehospital environment are needed. Logistical delivery issues also exist for BiPAP, and there is currently less convincing evidence of its safety in this setting. Emerging diagnostic assays and tools offer promise of fast and accurate diagnosis of CHF. Finally, transport of APE patients should be matched with the cardiovascular care resources of receiving facilities to optimize chances of survival.

ACKNOWLEDGMENT

Portions of this chapter are reprinted with the permission of the National Association of EMS Physicians from Mosesso VN Jr, Dunford J, Blackwell T, Griswell JK. Prehospital therapy for acute congestive heart failure: state of the art. *Prehosp Emerg Care* 2003;7:13–23.

REFERENCES

1. Nohria A, Lewis E, Stevenson LW. Medical management of advanced heart failure. *JAMA* 2002;287:628–640.
2. Croft JB, Giles WH, Pollard RA, et al. Heart failure survival among older adults in the United States: a poor prognosis for an emerging epidemic in the Medicare population. *Arch Intern Med* 1999;159:505–510.
3. Hunt SA, Baker DW, Chin MH, et al. ACC/AHA guidelines for the evaluation and management of chronic heart failure in the adult: executive summary. A report of the American College of Cardiology/American Heart Association Task Force on Practice Guidelines (Committee to revise the 1995 Guidelines for the Evaluation and Management of Heart Failure). *J Am Coll Cardiol* 2001;38:2101–2113.
4. Cotter G, Moshkovitz Y, Milovanov O, et al. Acute heart failure: a novel approach to its pathogenesis and treatment. *Eur J Heart Failure* 2002;4:227–234.
5. Gardtman M, Waagstein L, Karlsson T, Herlitz J. Has an intensified treatment in the ambulance of patients with acute severe left heart failure improved the outcome? *Eur J Emerg Med* 2000;7:15–24.
6. Bertini G, Giglioli C, Biggeri A, et al. Intravenous nitrates in the prehospital management of acute pulmonary edema. *Ann Emerg Med* 1997;30:493–499.
7. Guntupalli KK. Acute pulmonary edema. *Cardiol Clin* 1984;2:183–200.
8. Goldman. *Cecil textbook of medicine*, 21st ed. Philadelphia: WB Saunders, 2000.
9. Hoffman JR, Reynolds S. Comparison of nitroglycerin, morphine and furosemide in treatment of presumed prehospital pulmonary edema. *Chest* 1987; 92:586–593.
10. Kosowsky JM, Stephanides SL, Branson RD, Sayre MR. Prehospital use of continuous positive airway pressure (CPAP) for presumed pulmonary edema: a preliminary case series. *Prehosp Emerg Care* 2001;5:190–196.
11. Sacchetti AD, Harris RH. Acute cardiogenic pulmonary edema. What's the latest in emergency treatment? *Postgrad Med* 1998;103:145–147.
12. Cotter G, Kaluski E, Moshkovitz Y, et al. Pulmonary edema: new insight on pathogenesis and treatment. *Curr Opin Cardiol* 2001;16:159–163.
13. Mulrow C, Lucey C, Farnett L. Discriminating causes of dyspnea through the clinical examination. *J Gen Intern Med* 1993;8:383–392.
14. Schmitt B, Kushner M, Wiener S. The diagnostic usefulness of history of the patient with dyspnea. *J Gen Intern Med* 1986;1:386–393.
15. Little B, Ho KJ, Scott L. Electrocardiogram and rhythm strip interpretation by final year medical students. *Ulster Med J* 2001;70:108–110.
16. Marcus GM, Gerger IL, McKeown BH, et al. Association between phonocardiographic third and fourth heart sounds and objective measures of left ventricular function. *JAMA* 2005;293:2238–2244.
17. Peacock WF, Collins SP, Linsdsell CJ, et al. Gender and heart sounds in decompensated heart failure. *Acad Emerg Med* 2005;12(5):55(abst).
18. Maisel AS, Krishnaswamy P, Nowak RM, et al. Rapid measurement of B-type natriuretic peptide in the emergency diagnosis of heart failure. *N Engl J Med* 2002;347:161–167.

19. Maisel A. B-type natriuretic peptide in the diagnosis and management of congestive heart failure. *Cardiol Clin* 2001;19:557–571.

20. Dao Q, Krishnaswamy P, Kazanegra R, et al. Utility of B-type natriuretic peptide in the diagnosis of congestive heart failure in an urgent-care setting. *J Am Coll Cardiol* 2001;37:379–385.

21. Morrison LK, Harrison A, Krishnaswamy P, et al. Utility of a rapid B-natriuretic peptide assay in differentiating congestive heart failure from lung disease in patients presenting with dyspnea. *J Am Coll Cardiol* 2002;39:202–209.

22. Tabbibizar R, Maisel A. The impact of B-type natriuretic peptide levels on the diagnoses and management of congestive heart failure. *Curr Opin Cardiol* 2002;17:340–345.

23. Lee SC, Stevens TL, Sandberg SM, et al. The potential of brain natriuretic peptide as a biomarker for New York Heart Association class during the outpatient treatment of heart failure. *J Card Fail* 2002; 8:149–154.

24. Teboul A, Gaffinel A, Meune C, et al. Management of acute dyspnea: use and feasibility of brain natriuretic peptide (BNP) assay in the prehospital setting. *Resuscitation* 2004;61:91–96.

25. Marx J, Hockberger R, Walls R. *Rosen's emergency medicine: concepts and clinical practice*, 5th ed. St. Louis: Mosby, 2002.

26. Ventura HO, Pranulis MF, Young C, Smart FW. Impedance cardiography: a bridge between research and clinical practice in the treatment of heart failure. *Congest Heart Fail* 2000;6:94–102.

27. Kukovetz WR, Holzmann S. Mechanisms of nitrate-induced vasodilation and tolerance. *Eur J Clin Pharmacol* 1990;38:9.

28. Sacchetti A, Ramoska E, Moakes ME, et al. Effect of ED management on ICU use in acute pulmonary edema. *Am J Emerg Med* 1999,7.571–574.

29. Packer M. Neurohormonal interactions and adaptations in congestive heart failure. *Circulation* 1988;77:721.

30. Cotter G, Metzkor E, Kaluski E, et al. Randomised trial of high-dose isosorbide dinitrate plus low-dose furosemide versus high-dose furosemide plus low-dose isosorbide dinitrate in severe pulmonary oedema. *Lancet* 1998;351:389–393.

31. Wuerz R, Swope G, Meador S, et al. Safety of prehospital nitroglycerin. *Ann Emerg Med* 1994;23:31–36.

32. Northridge D. Frusemide or nitrates for acute heart failure? *Lancet* 1996;347:667–668.

33. Leeman M, Deguate JP. Invasive hemodynamic evaluation of sublingual captopril and nifedipine in patients with arterial hypertension after abdominal aortic surgery. *Crit Care Med* 1995;23:847.

34. Barnett J, Zink KM, Touchon RC. Sublingual captopril in the treatment of acute heart failure. *Curr Ther Res* 1991;49:274–281.

35. Hamilton RJ, Carter WA, Gallagher EJ. Rapid improvement of acute pulmonary edema with sublingual captopril. *Acad Emerg Med* 1996;3:205–212.

36. Ahmed A. Interaction between aspirin and angiotensin-converting enzyme inhibitors: should they be used together in older adults with heart failure? *J Am Geriatr Soc* 2002;50:1293–1296.

37. Annane D, Bellissant E, Pussard E, et al. Placebo-controlled, randomized, double-blind study of intravenous enalaprilat efficacy and safety in acute cardiogenic pulmonary edema. *Circulation* 1996;94:1316–1324.

38. Podbregar M, Voga G, Horvat M, et al. Bolus versus continuous low dose of enalaprilat in congestive heart failure with acute refractory decompensation. *Cardiology* 1999;91:41–49.

39. Colucci WS. Nesiritide for the treatment of decompensated heart failure. *J Card Fail* 2001;7:92–100.

40. Pingleton SK. Complications of acute respiratory failure. *Am Rev Respir Dis* 1988; 137:1463–1493.

41. Colice GL, Stukel TA, Dain B. Laryngeal complications of prolonged intubation. *Chest* 1989;96:877–884.

42. Craven DE, Steger KA. Epidemiology of nosocomial pneumonia: new perspectives on an old disease. *Chest* 1995;108:1S–16S.

43. Schnapp LM, Chin DP, Szaflarski N, et al. Frequency and importance of barotrauma in 100 patients with acute lung injury. *Crit Care Med* 1995;23:272–278.

44. Meduri GU, Turner RE, Abou-Shala N. Noninvasive positive pressure ventilation via face mask: first-line intervention in patients with acute hypercapnic and hypoxemic respiratory failure. *Chest* 1996;109:179–193.

45. Brochard L, Mancebo J, Wysocki M, et al. Noninvasive ventilation for acute exacerbations of chronic obstructive pulmonary disease. *N Engl J Med* 1995;333:817–822.

46. Bernstein AD, Holt AW, Vedig AE, et al. Treatment of severe cardiogenic pulmonary edema with continuous positive airway pressure delivered by face mask. *N Engl J Med* 1991;325:1825–1830.

47. Kramer N, Meyer TJ, Meharg J, et al. Randomized, prospective trial of noninvasive positive pressure ventilation in acute respiratory failure. *Am J Respir Crit Care Med* 1995;151:1799–1806.

48. Meduri GU, Cook TR, Turner RE, et al. Noninvasive positive pressure ventilation in status asthmaticus. *Chest* 1996;110:767–774.

49. Meduri GU, Conoscenti CC, Menashe P, et al. Noninvasive face mask ventilation in patients with acute respiratory failure. *Chest* 1989;95:865–870.

50. Pennock BE, Crashaw L, Kaplan PD. Noninvasive nasal mask ventilation for acute respiratory failure: institution of a new therapeutic technology for routine use. *Chest* 1994;105:441–444.

51. Baratz DM, Westbrook PR, Shah PK, et al. Effect of nasal continuous positive airway pressure on cardiac output and oxygen delivery in patients with congestive heart failure. *Chest* 1992;102:1397–1401.

52. Takeda S, Nejima J, Takano T, et al. Effect of nasal continuous positive airway pressure on pulmonary edema complicating acute myocardial infarction. *Jpn Circ J* 1998;62:553–558.

53. Kelly AM, Georgakas C, Bau S, Rosengarten P. Experience with the use of continuous positive airway pressure (CPAP) therapy in the emergency management of acute severe cardiogenic pulmonary oedema. *Aust N Z J Med* 1997;27:319–322.

54. Keenan SP, Kernerman PD, Cook DJ, et al. Effect of noninvasive positive pressure ventilation on mortality in patients admitted with acute respiratory failure: a meta-analysis. *Crit Care Med* 1997;25:1685–1692.

55. Pang D, Keenan SP, Cook DJ, Sibbald WJ. The effect of positive pressure airway support on mortality and the need for intubation in cardiogenic pulmonary edema: a systematic review. *Chest* 1998;114:1185–1192.

56. Mehta S, Jay GD, Woolard RH, et al. Randomized, prospective trial of bilevel versus continuous positive airway pressure in acute pulmonary edema. *Crit Care Med* 1997;25:620–628.

57. Masip J, Betbese AJ, Paez J, et al. Non-invasive pressure support ventilation versus conventional oxygen therapy in acute cardiogenic pulmonary oedema: a randomised trial. *Lancet* 2000;356:2126–2132.

OBSERVATION UNIT ADMISSION INCLUSION AND EXCLUSION CRITERIA

Sean P. Collins

BACKGROUND

Heart failure (HF) is a disease of epidemic proportions. Hospitalization accounts for the largest expenditure for care; annual costs are estimated to be $27.9 billion per year, about 3% of the total national health care budget.[1-3] In-hospital mortality ranges from 2% to 20% and 90-day recidivism in those discharged directly from the emergency department (ED) has been reported to be 61%.[4,5] Current guidelines for disposition are based on little or no empirical evidence.[6-8] As a direct result of the high-risk features of these patients and a lack of disposition guidance, the emergency physician's triage decisions are historically conservative; more than 80% of ED patients with acute decompensated heart failure (ADHF) are admitted to the hospital.[9] It has been suggested that poor ED risk stratification, particularly overestimation of disease severity, is the fundamental cause of the overutilization of limited in-hospital resources for this rapidly growing patient population.[10]

A novel approach for ADHF is necessary to decrease the relative burden of this disease. Despite recent advances in diagnostic and therapeutic measures for HF, the admission rate has remained largely unchanged. The observation unit (OU) presents an opportunity for further risk stratification and treatment for up to 24 hours to better delineate the need for admission. Using the OU to avoid hospital admission (average cost $5,456 per admission[3]) in just a small percentage of patients is likely to have a profound effect on health care expenditures.

The evaluation and disposition of ED patients with ADHF resembles the approach to chest pain in the 1980s, prior to the advent of chest pain centers. As a result of extensive research over the last 2 decades, we have experienced a dramatic paradigm shift in ED chest pain patients: from a high proportion of admitted patients to a rapid OU protocol allowing further risk stratification and safe, early discharge.[11-13] Preliminary research suggests a similar approach to ADHF may yield similar results.[14,15]

OBSERVATION UNIT MANAGEMENT OF ACUTE DECOMPENSATED HEART FAILURE

It has been suggested that appropriate candidates for the OU are those who have an expectation of (a) hospital stays less than 48 hours, (b) no diagnosis traditionally requiring hospitalization, (c) no procedure requiring hospitalization, and (d) no probability of death.[16] Due to the multiple comorbidities of ADHF patients, identifying a cohort that will fulfill these criteria is inherently difficult. However, excluding subjects with high-risk features,[5,17-23] as well as including subjects identified as proper candidates from previous OU research,[15,24,25] lends some guidance in patient selection. Our OU protocol is a collaborative effort between the Department of Emergency Medicine and the Division of Cardiology at the University of Cincinnati. Inclusion and exclusion criteria were selected based on a review of previously derived retrospective risk data and an OU protocol, so as to identify what current practice suggests is a low- to moderate-risk patient (Table 3–1).[5,15,17-23]

Inclusion Criteria

An ED diagnosis of HF is often based on history and physical examination findings along with ancillary tests such as chest radiography and electrocardiography. Distinguishing between cardiac and noncardiac causes of dyspnea by relying solely on these tests is difficult. The etiology is often determined after hospital admission based on right heart catheterization results or indirect measurement of ejection fraction via radionuclide scanning or echocardiography. The use of these tests to determine OU inclusion is not practical because they are not routinely available in EDs and their cost is prohibitive for use as a standardized screening test.

However, with an ED diagnosis of ADHF we also require patients to fulfill a modification of the Framingham criteria (Table 3–2). The Framingham criteria, reported in 1971, is one of the tools used to predict HF.[26,27] They were developed by following the natural history of HF over a 16-year period in more than 5,000 persons initially free of the disease. This tool uses "major" and "minor" criteria based on history, physical examination, and ancillary tests to categorize patients as definite, probable, and questionable HF. The Framingham criteria are well known for providing a useful probabilistic diagnosis of HF, and they are accepted criteria for establishing an etiology of dyspnea before definitive studies have been performed.[28] Furthermore, fulfillment of the Framingham criteria has not been shown to correlate with an increased risk of subsequent adverse events.[29] Four of the Framingham criteria are not used as part of our modified criteria: (a) circulation time, (b) vital capacity, (c) weight loss in response to treatment, and (d) autopsy findings. Vital capacity and circulation time are two parameters that are not measured in the ED, and weight loss in response to treatment would only help with a retrospective diagnosis of HF. Inclusion of patients requires two major or one major and two minor criteria.

TABLE 3–1 Inclusion and Exclusion Criteria for ADHF OU Management

Inclusion Criteria	Exclusion Criteria
Two from the left column OR one from the left column plus two from the right column[a] • Paroxysmal nocturnal dyspnea • Extremity edema • Neck vein distention • Night cough • Pulmonary edema (on CXR) • Dyspnea on exertion • Rales • Hepatomegaly • Cardiomegaly • Pleural effusion • S_3 gallop • Tachycardia ($\geq$130 beats/min) • Jugular venous distention • Positive hepatojugular reflex AND • Designated for admission by the emergency physician	• Alternative diagnosis explaining acute clinical presentation • Hypoxia (oxygen saturation <90% on room air) • Severe respiratory distress • Hypotension (systolic BP <90 mm Hg) • Temperature >100.0°F • Syncope • Requirement of intravenous infusion to treat hypotension or hypertension • Electrocardiogram with ischemic changes not known to be old • Serum markers indicative of myocardial necrosis • Severe electrolyte imbalances • Patients currently receiving dialysis • BNP <100 pg/mL

ADHF, acute decompensated heart failure; BNP, B-type natriuretic peptide; BP, blood pressure; CXR, chest x-ray; OU, observation unit.
[a]Adapted for emergency department use from the Framingham criteria.

TABLE 3–2 The Modified Framingham Criteria

Major	Minor
• Paroxysmal nocturnal dyspnea • Neck vein distention • Pulmonary edema (on CXR) • Rales • Cardiomegaly • S_3 gallop • Jugular venous distention • Positive hepatojugular reflex	• Extremity edema • Night cough • Dyspnea on exertion • Hepatomegaly • Pleural effusion • Tachycardia ($\geq$130 beats/min)

Exclusion Criteria

Patients are excluded for OU HF management if they have a feature that defines them as high risk (positive cardiac markers, systolic blood pressure <90 mm Hg) or have a concomitant illness that will make their discharge from the OU difficult (urgent need for dialysis, alternative diagnosis contributing to concurrent decompensation such as pneumonia). Based on its high sensitivity, a B-type natriuretic peptide (BNP) value less than 100 pg/mL is also used to exclude patients who are likely to not have AHDF as the underlying cause of their symptoms. Patients with new-onset ADHF can be managed in the OU; however, a facilitated workup will be needed as an outpatient.

PRELIMINARY RESULTS

We have been enrolling patients in our OU since May 2003 using the criteria listed in Table 3–1. Preliminary findings suggest it is safe and conserves hospital resources.[14] We conducted an observational, sequential cohort study. Both cohorts satisfied the inclusion and exclusion criteria identified in Table 3–1. During enrollment of the first cohort, the OU was not operational, whereas in the second group the OU was available to treating physicians. The first cohort of 36 ED patients was enrolled from April 2002 to April 2003 and the second group of 28 ED patients was enrolled from May 2003 to September 2003. With the exception of heart rate (90 vs. 99 beats per minute, $p = 0.02$) the patients were similar with regard to demographics and presenting vital signs ($p > 0.10$). Twenty percent of the first cohort was discharged from the ED, whereas 40% of the second cohort was discharged home after an OU stay. All patients in the first cohort were admitted to the hospital, whereas only 25% of patients in the second cohort were admitted to the hospital after an OU stay.

CONCLUSIONS

The OU represents an attractive alternative for further treatment and risk stratification of low- to medium-risk patients with ADHF. Safely avoiding hospitalization in a subset of patients is likely to result in a significant decrease in resource consumption. Current inclusion and exclusion criteria are based on what previous research has suggested are high-risk features in admitted patients, as well as on preliminary results of select OU protocols. Further prospective studies are needed to better characterize the safety and cost-effectiveness of the OU when compared with standard inpatient care.

REFERENCES

1. O'Connell JB BM. Economic impact of heart failure in the United States: a time for a different approach. *J Heart Lung Trans* 1994;13:S107–S112.
2. Stevenson LW, Braunwald E. Recognition and management of patients with heart failure. In: Goldman L, Braunwald E, eds. *Primary cardiology.* Philadelphia: WB Saunders, 1998: 310–329.

3. American Heart Association. *Heart disease and stroke statistics 2005 update.* Dallas, TX, 2004.

4. Fonarow GC, Adams KF Jr, Abraham WT, et al. Risk stratification for in-hospital mortality in acutely decompensated heart failure: classification and regression tree analysis. *JAMA* 2005;293:572–580.

5. Rame JE, Sheffield MA, Dries DL, et al. Outcomes after emergency department discharge with a primary diagnosis of heart failure. *Am Heart J* 2001;142:714–719.

6. Hunt SA, Abraham WT, Chin MH, et al. ACC/AHA 2005 guideline update for the diagnosis and management of chronic heart failure in the adult—summary article. A report of the American College of Cardiology/American Heart Association Task Force on Practice Guidelines (Writing Committee to Update the 2001 Guidelines for the Evaluation and Management of Heart Failure). *J Am Coll Cardiol* 2005;46:1116–1143.

7. HFSA guidelines for the management of patients with heart failure due to left ventricular systolic dysfunction pharmacological approaches. *Congest Heart Fail* 2000;6(1):11–39.

8. Konstam M, Dracup K, Baker D. Clinical Practice Guidelines No 11: heart failure: evaluation and care of patients with left-ventricular systolic dysfunction. Rockville, MD: Agency for Health Care Policy and Research 1994;94(0612).

9. Graff L, Orledge J, Radford MJ, et al. Correlation of the Agency for Health Care Policy and Research congestive heart failure admission guideline with mortality: peer review organization voluntary hospital association initiative to decrease events (PROVIDE) for congestive heart failure. *Ann Emerg Med* 1999;34(4 Pt 1):429–437.

10. Smith WR, Poses RM, McClish DK, et al. Prognostic judgments and triage decisions for patients with acute congestive heart failure. *Chest* 2002;121:1610–1617.

11. Tatum JL, Jesse RL, Kontos MC, et al. Comprehensive strategy for the evaluation and triage of the chest pain patient. *Ann Emerg Med* 1997;29:116–125.

12. Gibler WB, Runyon JP, Levy RC, et al. A rapid diagnostic and treatment center for patients with chest pain in the emergency department. *Ann Emerg Med* 1995;25:1–8.

13. Storrow AB, Gibler WB. Chest pain centers: diagnosis of acute coronary syndromes. *Ann Emerg Med* 2000;35:449–461.

14. Storrow AB, Collins SP, Lyons MS, et al. Emergency department observation of heart failure: preliminary analysis of safety and cost. *Congest Heart Fail* 2005;March–April:68–72.

15. Peacock WFT, Remer EE, Aponte J, et al. Effective observation unit treatment of decompensated heart failure. *Congest Heart Fail* 2002;8(2):68–73.

16. Sinclair D, Green R. Emergency department observation unit: can it be funded through reduced inpatient admission? *Ann Emerg Med* 1998;32:670–675.

17. Butler J, Hanumanthu S, Chomsky D, Wilson JR. Frequency of low-risk hospital admissions for heart failure. *Am J Cardiol* 1998;81:41–44.

18. Chin MH, Goldman L. Correlates of major complications or death in patients admitted to the hospital with congestive heart failure. *Arch Intern Med* 1996;156:1814–1820.

19. Chin MH, Goldman L. Correlates of early hospital readmission or death in patients with congestive heart failure. *Am J Cardiol* 1997;79:1640–1644.

20. Villacorta H, Rocha N, Cardoso R, et al. Hospital outcome and short-term follow-up of elderly patients presenting to the emergency unit with congestive heart failure. *Arq Bras Cardiol* 1998;70(3):167–171.

21. Selker HP, Griffith JL, D'Agostino RB. A time-insensitive predictive instrument for acute hospital mortality due to congestive heart failure: development, testing, and use for comparing hospitals: a multicenter study. *Med Care* 1994;32:1040–1052.

22. Esdaile JM, Horwitz RI, Levinton C, et al. Response to initial therapy and new onset as predictors of prognosis in patients hospitalized with congestive heart failure. *Clin Invest Med* 1992;15(2):122–131.

23. Katz MH, Nicholson BW, Singer DE, et al. The triage decision in pulmonary edema. *J Gen Intern Med* 1988;3:533–539.

24. Peacock WF, Young J, Collins SP, et al. Heart failure observation units: optimizing care. *Ann Emerg Med* 2006;47:22–32.

25. Peacock WF, Albert NM. Observation unit management of heart failure. *Emerg Med Clin North Am* 2001;19:209–232.

26. Ho KK, Anderson KM, Kannel WB, et al. Survival after the onset of congestive heart failure in Framingham Heart Study subjects. *Circulation* 1993;88:107–115.

27. McKee PA, Castelli WP, McNamara PM, Kannel WB. The natural history of congestive heart failure: the Framingham study. *N Engl J Med* 1971;285:1441–1446.

28. Di Bari M, Pozzi C, Cavallini MC, et al. The diagnosis of heart failure in the community. Comparative validation of four sets of criteria in unselected older adults: the ICARe Dicomano Study. *J Am Coll Cardiol* 2004;44:1601–1608.

29. Schellenbaum GD, Rea TD, Heckbert SR, et al. Survival associated with two sets of diagnostic criteria for congestive heart failure. *Am J Epidemiol* 2004;160:628–635.

4

ACUTE EXACERBATIONS OF HEART FAILURE: INITIAL EVALUATION AND MANAGEMENT IN THE ACUTE CARE SETTING

Douglas S. Ander

INTRODUCTION

Heart failure (HF) is a common diagnosis, facing approximately 4,900,000 people.[1] Over the past 3 decades we have seen a significant rise in the number of hospital discharges for HF,[1] and because the majority of admitted patients enter through the emergency department (ED),[2] proper initial management is important. Several studies on the use of the B-type natriuretic peptide (BNP) assay have indicated that earlier treatment in the ED can significantly impact hospital length of stay and cost.[3]

Patients may present to the ED with minimal symptoms, such as mild dyspnea or weight gain. Conversely, they may present to the ED with overt pulmonary edema. In addition to their fluid status, evaluation for adequate perfusion or evidence of shock should be considered. Recognition that HF patients may fall into different hemodynamic categories allows the clinician to tailor treatment based on the initial assessment. Using components of the history and physical examination, the clinician can develop a treatment plan individualized to that patient. Diuretics, vasodilators, angiotensin-converting enzyme inhibitors (ACEI), noninvasive ventilation, and natriuretic peptides can be used for hemodynamic and symptomatic needs.

Because of improvements in the treatment of HF that have resulted in improved survival, the emergency physician will see increased instances of acute exacerbations of HF. This chapter provides the reader with an understanding of the principles of initial acute HF management and examine specific therapeutic agents.

INITIAL STABILIZATION

The first step when a patient presents with presumed HF is to stabilize the clinical condition. This is followed by an evaluation including laboratory tests, radiographs, consideration of advance directives, and a search for reversible causes including ischemia and arrhythmias. Finally, treatment is instituted based on an assessment of the hemodynamic status.

Patients presenting with presumed HF should be initially assessed and stabilized. Those with impending respiratory failure should be treated with supplemental oxygen and the physician should consider the use of noninvasive ventilation. Patients who are unable to control their airway, cannot tolerate noninvasive ventilation, or worsen despite these measures should be considered for endotracheal intubation.

When HF is considered the most likely etiology of the patient's symptoms, the initial workup should include establishment of intravenous (IV) access, a focused history and physical examination, assessment of the degree of fluid overload and perfusion, evaluation of oxygenation, assessment of the cardiac rhythm, evaluation for cardiac ischemia with a 12-lead electrocardiogram, and a chest radiography. Blood work should be based on clinical suspicion and may include a complete blood cell count, electrolytes, BNP or N-terminal pro-BNP levels, and cardiac markers.

Advance directives should be discussed with the patient or family, especially in those with severe exacerbations of chronic disease. This information will help direct the management plan.

The clinician should look for precipitants of the HF (Table 4–1). The identifiable reversible causes should be treated in conjunction with the treatment of the HF. Unfortunately, in one study the authors could not identify a precipitant in 40% of the HF presentations.[4] Patient-related factors such as noncompliance with medication and diet should be addressed. In several studies, poor compliance was the precipitant of the acute exacerbation, ranging from 21% to 41.9%.[4,5] Patient and family education cannot be underestimated. Several studies have investigated the impact of education and find that it significantly decreases hospital readmissions.[6-8]

Cardiac ischemia is a leading cause of HF and an important cause of acute exacerbation.[9] Although not every exacerbation of chronic HF will require a workup of an ischemic etiology, the clinician should be aware of the potential and consider it accordingly. Cardiac arrhythmias are associated with a worse prognosis in HF.[10] In the acute care setting, cardiac arrhythmias such as atrial fibrillation, ventricular arrhythmias, and conduction abnormalities can be precipitants of exacerbations. Treatment should be focused on the hemodynamic effects and not correction of every arrhythmia. Patients with chronic HF are at significant risk for ventricular arrhythmias.

PRINCIPLES OF TREATMENT

The classic picture of an HF patient with acute pulmonary edema frothing at the mouth and appearing cyanotic is only one possible presentation. Some individuals present with respiratory distress, but others may have

TABLE 4–1 **Precipitants of Heart Failure Exacerbations**

Noncompliance
    Medications
    Diet
Ischemic events
        Acute myocardial infarction
        Cardiac ischemia
Uncontrolled hypertension
Valvular disease
Cardiac arrhythmias
        Atrial fibrillation with a rapid ventricular response
        Ventricular tachycardia
        Bradycardia
        Conduction abnormalities
Noncardiac events
        Pulmonary embolus
        Anemia
        Systemic infection (e.g., urosepsis,. pneumonia)
        Thyroid disorders
        Stress
        Drugs and alcohol
Adverse effects of medications

only mild symptomatic dyspnea and others have only fatigue. Some present hypotensive and others with significant hypertension.

Categorizing HF patients using a hemodynamic classification system (Figure 4–1) is a useful approach. Based on the initial history and physical examination, patients can be placed into a hemodynamic category and then appropriate therapy can be selected. Fluid overload can be assessed by the presence or absence of dyspnea, orthopnea, pulmonary rales, elevated jugular venous pressure, the presence of a third heart sound S_3, and hepatomegaly. Perfusion can be estimated by evaluating for the presence or absence of fatigue, nausea, symptomatic hypotension, and cool extremities (Table 4–2).

The physician must recognize that these signs and symptoms can be inaccurate and have a low inter-rater reliability.[11] Assessment using these historical and physical diagnostic clues needs to be considered in aggregate and supplemented with more objective diagnostic testing (chest radiograph, BNP or pro-BNP level, bioimpedance measurements, digital S_3 detection) to improve accuracy. At this point, this clinical assessment strategy provides the best estimate of the patient's hemodynamic status.

		Congestion at rest	
		No	Yes
Low perfusion at rest	No	Warm and Dry A	Warm and Wet B
	Yes	Cold and Dry D	Cold and Wet C

FIGURE 4-1 Bedside assessment of hemodynamic status and corresponding therapeutic intervention. (Adapted from Stevenson et al.)

A: Well compensated. If symptomatic typically require minor adjustments in medications and follow-up.
B: Fluid overloaded and well perfused. Vasodilators and diuretics are the treatment modalities.
C: Diminished perfusion and fluid overloaded. For those with elevated SVR, vasodilators and diuretics should improve cardiac output. Inotropic support for low blood pressure may be required.
D: Poor perfusion and dry. Typically require a fluid bolus. Consider the addition of inotropic support for patients unresponsive to the initial bolus.

Most patients presenting with HF are fluid overloaded but have adequate perfusion, that is, "wet and warm." These patients require diuretics and vasodilation. The fluid-overloaded patient could also present with diminished perfusion, called "wet and cold." Those with elevated systemic vascular resistance (SVR) will require vasodilation. Those with symptomatic hypotension and diminished SVR may require inotropic support. The least common patient is the patient that has been overdiuresed and has evidence of hypoperfusion, the "dry and cold." If manifesting symptomatic hypotension, this patient may require a fluid bolus and the addition of inotropic support. As a guiding principle, chronic HF patients are best served by lower blood pressures, with a systolic blood pressure as low as 80 to 90 mm Hg. As long as they are asymptomatic, continue to mentate, and have appropriate urine output, no further blood pressure treatment is necessary.

**TABLE 4–2   Clinical Bedside Assessment
of Heart Failure**

Evidence of congestion
Dyspnea
Orthopnea
Paroxysmal nocturnal dyspnea
Jugular venous distention
Hepatojugular reflex
Third heart sound
Edema
Hepatomegaly
Rales
Evidence of diminished perfusion
Fatigue
Nausea
Narrow pulse pressure
Cool extremities
Symptomatic hypotension
(asymptomatic, continue to mentate, and have appropriate urine output)

This hemodynamic classification system provides the physician with a framework for the initial assessment and treatment of the HF patient. However, this framework is based on imprecise measures; therefore, the initial treatment must be guided by good clinical judgment and must be adjusted depending on the initial response to the therapeutic interventions. Until better and more accurate diagnostic modalities are available, the physician should use the framework presented in this section to develop the therapeutic plan.

SPECIFIC THERAPEUTIC AGENTS AND MODALITIES

Diuretics

Patients presenting with evidence of fluid overload, the "wet" patient, benefit by the use of a diuretic. Loop diuretics act through the inhibition of sodium reabsorption at the loop of Henle to promote diuresis. The resultant volume reduction causes a decrease in filling pressures and pulmonary congestion. This provides the patient with symptomatic improvement. Peak diuretic effect is typically seen within 30 minutes of administration. Physicians should be aware that some studies have demonstrated adverse physiologic effects of furosemide administration including initial increases in filling pressures prior to diuresis and adverse neurohormonal effects by increasing renin, norepinephrine, and vasopressin levels.[12]

The usual starting dose of furosemide is 20 to 80 mg intravenously. A patient with no previous exposure to furosemide may have adequate response to lower doses. If a patient is currently on furosemide, using the current enteral dose as an IV bolus is a good starting point. If no response is seen within 30 to 60 minutes, the dose can be doubled. Treatment with diuretics may lead to hypokalemia and hypomagnesemia; therefore, monitoring and treatment of electrolyte abnormalities is important. Despite some of the potential hemodynamic and neurohormonal effects of loop diuretics, diuresis and symptomatic improvement seen with furosemide administration make it the drug of choice for the fluid-overloaded patient.

Nitrates

The patient with fluid overload and reasonable perfusion ("wet and warm") can be successfully treated with a reduction in preload, which decreases ventricular workload. Nitroglycerin (NTG) achieves the reduction in filling pressures by dilation of the venous system.[13] At higher doses, there is dilation of the arterial system, causing decreased left ventricular (LV) work. NTG also dilates epicardial coronary arteries, increasing collateral blood flow.[14] Some evidence exists showing that high doses of nitrates results in better outcomes, with decreased need for mechanical ventilation and fewer myocardial infarctions.[15,16] As long as there is adequate blood pressure, NTG can be administered sublingually as either a spray or a pill (0.4 mg) at 1-minute intervals. This can be done effectively before institution of IV access. This may be followed by transdermal NTG paste (1 to 2 inches), if the patient is perfusing adequately to permit absorption. If continued reductions in preload and afterload are required, an NTG drip may be started and titrated to effect. Dosing can start at 10 to 20 μg per minute and titrated quickly every 3 to 5 minutes. Doses can reach 200 to 300 μg per minute to achieve the desired effect. Adverse effects of nitrates include headache, sinus tachycardia, abdominal pain, tachyphylaxis, and hypotension. Despite a minimal number of prospective trials, nitrates with diuretics form the basis behind the treatment of the fluid-overloaded patient.

Nitroprusside

Some patients with extreme elevations of SVR require additional afterload reduction not provided by NTG. Nitroprusside (NTP) can be added if further afterload reduction is warranted. NTP is a potent vasodilator that relaxes both arteriolar and venous smooth muscle, with resultant improvement in cardiac output and stroke volume.[17] The decrease in preload and afterload results in augmentation of cardiac output and stroke volume. IV infusion dose starts at 0.1 to 0.2 μg/kg/minute and can be increased every 5 minutes. Dangerous hypotension can occur precipitously, mandating continuous blood pressure monitoring. Other adverse effects include the theoretic "coronary steal" syndrome if a fixed epicardial coronary artery obstruction exists. Patients with renal failure are at risk for thiocyanate toxicity with prolonged administration of NTP. Finally, a reflex tachycardia may adversely affect myocardial oxygen consumption.

Morphine

Morphine sulfate has potential hemodynamic benefits in the treatment of HF by causing an increase in venous capacitance and a decrease in preload.[18] Morphine is administered in incremental doses of 2 to 10 mg every 5 to 15 minutes. It should be titrated to effect with careful observation of its respiratory and hemodynamic effects. Patients with acute pulmonary edema present with significant air hunger. In this population, morphine has the ability to decrease anxiety and may be beneficial. Unfortunately, very limited data support the therapeutic advantages of using morphine. One retrospective study has associated morphine with an increased need for intensive care unit admission.[19]

Fluids

Patients with poor perfusion and who have been overdiuresed, the "cold and dry," typically report an increased use of their diuretics. They can be recognized by symptoms of increased fatigue, nausea, cool extremities, and hypotension, without any evidence of fluid overload. Although counterintuitive to the treatment of HF, these patients may benefit from a fluid bolus of 250 to 500 mL of isotonic fluid. This should be done cautiously with continuous reassessment of the patient's response and fluid status.

Inotropic/Pressor Support

In the patient with poor perfusion and signs of fluid overload, the "cool and wet," inotropic support is sometimes indicated. Vasodilators and diuretics are first-line agents, but if the patient does not have an adequate response and has evidence of poor perfusion without overt shock, pure beta agonists such as dobutamine or a phosphodiesterase inhibitor such as milrinone may be required. The initial dose of dobutamine is 2 to 5 μg/kg/minute, which can be titrated up to 20 μg/kg/minute. Dobutamine, as a beta-1 receptor agonist, acts to increase myocardial contractility and improve cardiac output. In most patients, this should be sufficient to overcome the vasodilator effects of the beta-2 activity. Caution should be exercised because, in patients with borderline hypotension, the addition of dobutamine may lead to significant hypotension.

If cardiogenic shock is present, a mixed catecholamine agonist such as dopamine may be added to the regimen. One should remember that cardiogenic shock implies evidence of poor perfusion and is not dependent on the blood pressure. Intra-aortic balloon pump placement may also be considered as a bridge to cardiac transplantation.

Natriuretic Peptides

The "warm and wet" patient, and even the patient with some degree of hypoperfusion, may benefit from vasodilation. Nesiritide (Scios, Tremont, CA) is an IV human BNP and provides a combination of neurohormonal and hemodynamic effects that may be beneficial in the initial management of HF. Neurohormonal effects include improved sodium and water excretion and decreased endothelin, norepinephrine, aldosterone, renin, and angiotensin levels.[20] Hemodynamic effects include decreasing filling pressures and SVR and an increase in cardiac output, without an increase in heart rate.[20-22]

Several trials have studied the effects of nesiritide on inpatients with HF. Colucci et al.[23] reported a dose-dependent decrease in filling pressures and improved symptoms. The Vasodilation in the Management of Acute HF trial compared the addition of IV nesiritide or IV NTG to standard HF therapy.[24] Nesiritide, administered as a 2 µg per kilogram bolus, followed by a maintenance infusion of 0.01 µg/kg/minute resulted in decreased filling pressures and improvement in dyspnea compared with standard therapy. In the observation unit, nesiritide is safe and its use resulted in decreased 30-day readmissions to the hospital as compared with standard therapy.[25]

Although no large-scale trials exist using nesiritide, it has comparable or slightly better hemodynamic attributes than NTG, does not need to be titrated, has no associated tachycardia or tachyphylaxis, is nonarrhythmogenic, and attenuates the neurohormonal derangements of HF. Based on two recent meta-analyses of nesiritide, clinicians should be cautious when instituting therapy.[26,27] Before starting nesiritide, there should be clear indications of decompensated HF in patients who have failed standard therapy. Future large studies are necessary to elucidate the best and safest use of nesiritide.

Angiotensin-Converting Enzyme Inhibitors

The renin-angiotensin-aldosterone system (RAAS) plays an important role in the neurohormonal derangements of HF. Activation of the RAAS, although initially beneficial, leads to many of the adverse hemodynamic consequences of HF. The ability of ACE inhibitors (ACEIs) to relax both arterial resistance and venous vessels and to lower impedance to LV ejection provides the patient with a hemodynamic advantage. Patients with asymptomatic LV dysfunction and chronic HF derive a mortality reduction from therapy with ACEI.[28,29] Several studies of severe chronic HF demonstrate dramatic improvements in hemodynamics immediately after administration of an ACEI.[30-32]

Some preliminary evidence exists supporting the use of an ACEI for acute exacerbations of HF.[33,34] In a small prospective, randomized, double-blind, placebo-controlled trial of 48 patients, Hamilton and Gallagher[34] evaluated the role of sublingual captopril for acute pulmonary edema. They measured HF severity using a composite of four parameters: patient-reported dyspnea, physician judgment of respiratory distress, diaphoresis, and level of bed elevation tolerance. Using this composite score, they demonstrated that sublingual captopril results in better scores during the first 40 minutes of therapy. However, there was no change in mortality, admissions, or intubation rates and this study was too small to evaluate safety.

ACEIs can be administered as captopril 25 mg by mouth or sublingually. Oral captopril has an onset of action within 15 to 30 minutes. Sublingual captopril decreases pulmonary capillary wedge pressure significantly after 10 minutes.[35] Captopril should probably be avoided if the patient's systolic blood pressure is less than 90 mm Hg.

Despite the lack of definitive, large-scale trials, some centers advocate the use ACEIs as a routine component of their therapeutic regimen.[19] Based on hemodynamic data and one ED study, addition of ACEIs in patients with high SVR appears to be advantageous. Because there are no large placebo-controlled trials using ACEIs in the acute care setting, their use cannot be recommended as a standard of care.

Respiratory Considerations

All patients presenting with HF should receive supplemental oxygen. Patients with respiratory distress and dyspnea will typically respond to aggressive medical management. Failure of medical management and worsening respiratory status may lead to endotracheal intubation. Two noninvasive ventilatory techniques are continuous positive airway pressure (CPAP) or bilevel positive airway pressure (BiPAP), which may be used to treat the respiratory distress.

CPAP, when added to standard therapy in HF patients, does not change overall hospital mortality[36–38] but does decrease endotracheal intubations. A pooled systematic review comparing standard therapy with and without CPAP reported a trend in the reduction of the risk of mortality of −6.6% (95% CI: −16% to +3%) and a reduction in the risk of intubation of −26% (95% CI: −13% to −38%).[39]

A pooled review comparing BiPAP to standard therapy revealed intubation rates for BiPAP ranging from 0% to 44% and mortality rates from 0% to 22%.[39] A more recent trial, not included in the pooled analysis, reported an intubation rate for BiPAP of 23.8% versus a 41.2% standard therapy rate.[40] In the BiPAP group, there was a lower myocardial infarction rate as compared with standard therapy, 19% versus 29.4%, respectively. Only one randomized trial has compared CPAP directly with BiPAP.[41] The researchers found no difference in hospital mortality or intubation rates. The study was halted early due to a high rate of myocardial infarction in the BiPAP group compared with the CPAP cohort, 71% versus 31%, $p = 0.006$, respectively. It is unclear whether this phenomenon is unique to the BiPAP or due to a higher number of patients in the BiPAP group with chest pain potentially indicating underlying ischemia.

Noninvasive ventilation to avoid endotracheal intubation has some promise in the treatment of severe respiratory distress. Data with large-scale studies is lacking, and some evidence even exists that noninvasive ventilation may be harmful. The clinician should use caution when considering the use of noninvasive ventilation in HF, especially in the patient with possible ischemic heart disease.

CONCLUSION

The management of patients with acute exacerbations of HF is difficult because the history, physical examination, and chest radiography lack the accuracy clinicians need to accurately make the diagnosis and determine the degree of decompensation. Clinicians must use the tools at hand in the acute care setting to accurately diagnose and categorize the hemodynamic derangements. Once the patient's clinical condition has been stabilized, he or she can be treated based on hemodynamic classification. Treatment should be focused on improving symptoms, decreasing volume overload, and improving perfusion. In the majority of cases, this can be done with diuretics and vasodilators. In some, the addition of inotropic agents and pressor agents may be needed to improve perfusion.

Ongoing research on the diagnosis, management, and disposition of patients presenting with ADHF is needed, especially in the acute care environment. Applying the results from research in chronic HF or from the inpatient cohort to the acute care population is fraught with potential for error. As this research grows, clinicians can expect to become more accurate in diagnosing HF and providing treatment specifically designed to combat the neurohormonal and hemodynamic changes of HF.

REFERENCES

1. American Heart Association. *Heart disease and stroke statistics–2005 update.* Dallas, TX: American Heart Association, 2005.

2. *ADHERE, Acute decompensated heart failure national registry,* Vol. 4th quarter 2002 National Database. Sunnyvale, CA: ADHERE, 2003.

3. Mueller C, et al. Use of B-type natriuretic peptide in the evaluation and management of acute dyspnea [see comment]. *N Engl J Med* 2004;350:647–654.

4. Opasich C, et al. Precipitating factors and decision-making processes of short-term worsening heart failure despite "optimal" treatment (from the IN-CHF Registry). *Am J Cardiol* 2001;88:382–387.

5. Michalsen A, Konig G, Thimme W. Preventable causative factors leading to hospital admission with decompensated heart failure [see comment]. *Heart* 1998;80:437–441.

6. Philbin EF. Comprehensive multidisciplinary programs for the management of patients with congestive heart failure [comment]. *J Gen Intern Med* 1999;14:130–135.

7. Rich MW, et al. A multidisciplinary intervention to prevent the readmission of elderly patients with congestive heart failure [comment]. *N Engl J Med* 1995;333:1190–1195.

8. West JA, et al. A comprehensive management system for heart failure improves clinical outcomes and reduces medical resource utilization. *Am J Cardiol* 1997;79:58–63.

9. Goldberger JJ, et al. Prognostic factors in acute pulmonary edema. *Arch Intern Med* 1986;146:489–493.

10. Drics DL, et al. Atrial fibrillation is associated with an increased risk for mortality and heart failure progression in patients with asymptomatic and symptomatic left ventricular systolic dysfunction: a retrospective analysis of the SOLVD trials. Studies of Left Ventricular Dysfunction. *J Am Coll Cardiol* 1998;32:695–703.

11. Badgett RG, Lucey CR, Mulrow CD. Can the clinical examination diagnose left-sided heart failure in adults? [see comments.]. *JAMA* 1997;277:1712–1719.

12. Francis GS, et al. Acute vasoconstrictor response to intravenous furosemide in patients with chronic congestive heart failure. Activation of the neurohumoral axis. *Ann Intern Med* 1985;103:1–6.

13. Bussmann WD, Schupp D. Effect of sublingual nitroglycerin in emergency treatment of severe pulmonary edema. *Am J Cardiol* 1978;41: 931–936.

14. Cohen MCDJ, Sonnenblick EH, Kirk ES. The effects of nitroglycerin on coronary collaterals and myocardial contractility. *J Clin Invest* 1973;52: 2836–2847.

15. Cotter G, et al. Randomised trial of high-dose isosorbide dinitrate plus low-dose furosemide versus high-dose furosemide plus low-dose isosorbide dinitrate in severe pulmonary oedema. *Lancet* 1998;351:389–393.

16. Sharon A, et al. High-dose intravenous isosorbide-dinitrate is safer and better than Bi-PAP ventilation combined with conventional treatment for severe pulmonary edema [comment]. *J Am Coll Cardiol* 2000;36:832–837.

17. Rossen RM, Alderman EL, Harrison DC. Circulatory response to vasodilator therapy in congestive cardiomyopathy. *Br Heart J* 1976;38:695–700.

18. Vismara LA, Leaman DM, Zelis R. The effects of morphine on venous tone in patients with acute pulmonary edema. *Circulation* 1976;54:335–337.

19. Sacchetti A, et al. Effect of ED management on ICU use in acute pulmonary edema. *Am J Emerg Med* 1999;17:571–574.

20. Abraham WT, et al. Systemic hemodynamic, neurohormonal, and renal effects of a steady-state infusion of human brain natriuretic peptide in patients with hemodynamically decompensated heart failure. *J Cardiac Fail* 1998;4:37–44.

21. Marcus LS, et al. Hemodynamic and renal excretory effects of human brain natriuretic peptide infusion in patients with congestive heart failure. A double-blind, placebo-controlled, randomized crossover trial. *Circulation* 1996;94:3184–3189.

22. Hobbs RE, et al. Hemodynamic effects of a single intravenous injection of synthetic human brain natriuretic peptide in patients with heart failure secondary to ischemic or idiopathic dilated cardiomyopathy. *Am J Cardiol* 1996;78:896–901.

23. Colucci WS, et al. Intravenous nesiritide, a natriuretic peptide, in the treatment of decompensated congestive heart failure. Nesiritide Study Group. *N Engl J Med* 2000;343: 246–253.

24. Publication Committee for the V.I. Intravenous nesiritide vs nitroglycerin for treatment of decompensated congestive heart failure: a randomized controlled trial. *JAMA* 2002;287:1531–1540.

25. Peacock WF 4th, Holland R, Gyarmathy R, et al. Observation unit treatment of heart failure with nesiritide: results from the proaction trial. *J Emerg Med* 2005;29: 243–252.

26. Sackner-Bernstein JD, Skopicki HA, Aaronson KD. Risk of worsening renal function with nesiritide in patients with acutely decompensated heart failure [see comment]. *Circulation* 2005;111:1487–1491.

27. Sackner-Bernstein JD, et al. Short-term risk of death after treatment with nesiritide for decompensated heart failure: a pooled analysis of randomized controlled trials. *JAMA* 2005;293:1900–1905.

28. Effects of enalapril on mortality in severe congestive heart failure. Results of the Cooperative North Scandinavian Enalapril Survival Study (CONSENSUS). The CONSENSUS Trial Study Group. *N Engl J Med* 1987;316:1429–1435.

29. Effect of enalapril on survival in patients with reduced left ventricular ejection fractions and congestive heart failure. The SOLVD Investigators. *N Engl J Med* 1991;325:293–302.

30. Haude M, Erbel R, Meyer J. Sublingual administration of captopril versus nitroglycerin in patients with severe congestive heart failure. *Int J Cardiol* 1990;27: 351–359.

31. Powers ER, Stone J, Reison DS, et al. The effect of captopril on renal, coronary, and systemic hemodynamics in patients with severe congestive heart failure. *Am Heart J* 1982;104:1203–1210.

32. Kubo SH, Laragh JH, Prida XE, et al. Immediate converting enzyme inhibition with intravenous enalapril in chronic congestive heart failure. *Am J Cardiol* 1985;55:122–126.

33. Annane D, et al. Placebo-controlled, randomized, double-blind study of intravenous enalaprilat efficacy and safety in acute cardiogenic pulmonary edema. *Circulation* 1996;94:1316–1324.

34. Hamilton RJ, Gallagher EJ. Rapid improvement of acute pulmonary edema with sublingual captopril. *Acad Emerg Med* 1996;3:205–212.

35. Barnett JC, Touchon RC. Sublingual captopril in the treatment of acute heart failure. *Curr Ther Res* 1991;49:274–281.

36. Bersten AD, et al. Treatment of severe cardiogenic pulmonary edema with continuous positive airway pressure delivered by face mask. *N Engl J Med* 1991;325:1825–1830.

37. Lin M, et al. Reappraisal of continuous positive airway pressure therapy in acute cardiogenic pulmonary edema. Short-term results and long-term follow-up. *Chest* 1995;107: 1379–1386.

38. Rasanen J, et al. Continuous positive airway pressure by face mask in acute cardiogenic pulmonary edema. *Am J Cardiol* 1985;55:296–300.

39. Pang D, et al. The effect of positive pressure airway support on mortality and the need for intubation in cardiogenic pulmonary edema: a systematic review. *Chest* 1998;114: 1185–1192.

40. Levitt MA. A prospective, randomized trial of BiPAP in severe acute congestive heart failure. *J Emerg Med* 2001;21:363–369.

41. Mehta S, et al. Randomized, prospective trial of bilevel versus continuous positive airway pressure in acute pulmonary edema. *Crit Care Med* 1997;25:620–628.

THE PROCESS AND ECONOMICS OF HEART FAILURE

Sandra Sieck

INTRODUCTION

Heart failure (HF) is the only cardiac disease whose incidence and prevalence are increasing, a trend that threatens to impose an exponentially increasing burden on the health care system.[1,2] This burden impacts patients, providers, insurers, health care suppliers, and particularly hospitals, where the majority of health care is rendered to those with acute decompensated heart failure (ADHF).

Much progress has been made in the clinical treatment of HF with aggressive pharmacologic and device therapies, but the difficulty in treating these patients effectively while maintaining a healthy balance of economic viability is the goal of the acute care facility. Defining and implementing optimal care that is cost-effective and results in best clinical outcomes, quality of life, and satisfaction of patient and providers has been a challenge to the health care delivery system. As advances in technology add increasing costs to the treatment of HF patients, reimbursements remain limited and place the onus on the acute care facility to ensure the provision of cost-efficient care while maintaining a high of quality of care. As the population ages, the health care system will be forced to develop more innovative approaches to the care and treatment of patients with chronic diseases that are prone to exacerbations resulting in costly health care utilization.

BURDEN OF DISEASE

HF is responsible for more elderly patient hospitalizations than any other disease.[1] High readmission rates—20% at 30 days and 50% at 6 months—also contribute to the staggering figure: a total of 6.5 million hospital days are expended to treat ADHF.[3] Hospital discharges for HF in 2001 were estimated to be approaching 1 million (Figure 5–1). In fact, HF is the most commonly used Medicare diagnosis-related group (DRG).[4] The high utilization not only is reflected in the inpatient sector, this diagnosis also accounts for 12 to 15 million office visits annually.[5] These utilization figures have continued on an increasing trend over the last 2 decades.

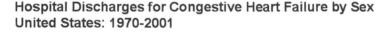

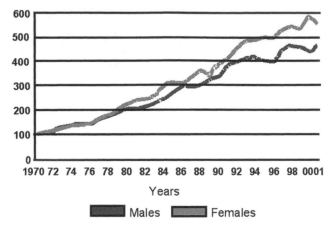

Note: Hospital discharges include people both living and dead.

Source: CDC/NCHS

FIGURE 5-1 Trends in U.S. hospital discharge rates. From American Heart Association 2004 Statistical Update, p. 24 (Fig. 2).

HF patients are considerably expensive patients as well and contributed to $25.8 billion in 2004 in direct and indirect costs to the United States.[6] Compared with other cardiac conditions, HF accounts for more than 10% of total costs for all cardiovascular conditions (Table 5-1). Although charges for medications, provider fees, and nursing care contribute to these costs, the majority of the expenditures are related to acute hospitalizations (Figure 5-2). These figures substantiate the large health care burden of HF, both clinically and financially. Although these figures represent high-level economic views, the overall burden can easily be translated to the level of the individual hospital.

CURRENT PRACTICES

Currently, the majority of ADHF patients are treated in the inpatient environment. The emergency department (ED) is the point of entry for three out of every four ADHF patients, and 75% to 90% of HF patients presenting to the ED are ultimately admitted to the hospital.[7,8] Once admitted to the hospital, the average length of stay (LOS) is 7.0 days.[9]

After the Balanced Budget Act of 1997 and the Refinement Act of 1999, hospitals began struggling and continue to struggle with the Inpatient Prospective Payment System (IPPS) and the Outpatient Prospective Payment System (OPPS). Most facilities are reimbursed for ADHF patients on a fixed inpatient payment under the DRG system and must operate with optimal efficiency to maintain financial viability.

TABLE 5–1   **Cardiovascular Disease Costs (in $billion) in the United States**

	Coronary Heart Disease	Hypertension	CHF	Total Cardiovascular Disease[a,b]
Direct costs				
Hospital	37.0	5.5	13.6	101.7
Nursing home	9.7	3.8	3.5	38.1
Physicians/other professionals	9.6	9.6	1.8	33.4
Drugs/other medical durables	8.5	21.0	2.7	43.3
Home health care	1.4	1.5	2.1	10.3
Total expenditures[b]	66.3	41.5	23.7	226.7
Indirect costs				
Lost productivity/morbidity	9.1	7.2	–	33.6
Lost productivity/mortality[c]	57.8	6.8	2.1	108.1
Grand totals[b]	133.2	55.5	25.8	368.4

CHF, congestive heart failure.
[a]Original table included stroke and heart disease, which are included in the total cardiovascular disease figures.
[b]Totals may not add up due to rounding and overlap.
[c]Lost future earnings of persons who will die in 2004, discounted at 3%.
Adapted from American Heart Association, American Stroke Association. Heart Disease and Stroke Statistics–2004 Update. Available at: http://www.americanheart.org/downloadable/heart/1079736729696 HDSStats2004UpdateREV3-19-04.pdf

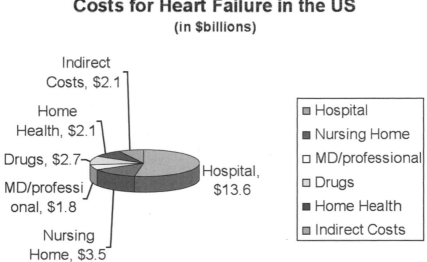

Costs for Heart Failure in the US
(in $billions)

FIGURE 5–2   Costs for heart failure in the United States. Data taken from Table 5–1.

Placement of the ADHF patient in an inpatient bed can easily consume the average Medicare payment of $4,617 currently reimbursed for DRG 127 under the IPPS. With an average LOS of more than 5 days combined with the break-even point for most hospitals occurring at about 5 days, most hospitals are not adequately reimbursed to cover these costs.[10] In a review of 2001 cost data, the average hospital lost $1,288 per ADHF patient.[10] Such losses obviously represent a serious impact on a hospital's operation and fiscal stability.

Another unique characteristic of reimbursement under Medicare affects the HF patient who has been recently discharged after an acute admission and is readmitted within 30 days. Nearly 20% of patients discharged from an acute hospitalization for exacerbation of congestive heart failure (CHF) are readmitted within 30 days, and 50% are readmitted within 6 months.[11,12] With repeat admissions within a 30-day period, payment is not guaranteed and potential audits could occur. Return visits create burden of proof on the facility with medical necessity to justify the return visit within 30 days. Medicare may not reimburse the hospital, and payment could be vulnerable at the expense of the facility. Because most HF patients are covered under Medicare, many hospitals are faced with a fiscal loss when rendering care to the ADHF patient under the current Medicare DRG reimbursement levels. The relative weight of DRG 127 (HF) is less than DRG 89 Pneumonia. Of course, the current practice patterns regarding inpatient admissions contribute to these fiscal problems. As hospitals are seeing increasingly ill patients, it is becoming more difficult to offset these losses by caring for other conditions. Therefore, acute care facilities are forced to find alternative solutions in providing quality care for ADHF in a fiscally sound manner.

EMERGENCE OF THE OBSERVATION UNIT

In general, efforts in health care delivery are moving in the direction of providing more services in the outpatient setting. Care in such settings is commonly less costly and more efficient. As an example, chest pain centers (CPCs) again began to emerge in the late 1990s for patients presenting with chest pain, as a more efficient way of ruling out myocardial infarction in low-risk patient subsets. The method proved not only more logistically efficient but more cost-effective as well.

The Centers for Medicare and Medicaid Services (CMS) have now targeted chest pain, asthma, and HF for efforts to reduce morbidity and mortality through use of intense treatment in nonacute care settings. This strategy, coupled with the positive experiences gained from the CPCs, has led to the emergence of the observation unit (OU), a service provided "on-hospital premises, including use of a bed and periodic monitoring by nursing or other staff, which are reasonable and necessary to evaluate an outpatient's condition or determine the need for possible admission as an inpatient."[13]

TABLE 5-2 Utilization of Observation Units

Year	Total Number of Observation Services	Total Patients for HF Observation Services
2002	30,094	1,603
2003	66,276	3,749

HF, heart failure.
From Utilization of Observation Units Medicare Outpatient Prospective Payment System
Data: Observation Services Claim Data (G244, G263), Scios Inc., data on file, 2004.

Use of the OU has dramatically increased over the last few years (Table 5-2). Between 2002 and 2003, there was an 85% increase in OU utilization. Chest pain represented the most common condition seen in an OU, followed by gastrointestinal disorders and asthma.[14] ADHF accounted for 5% of OU conditions in 2002 to 2003.

In April 2002, CMS developed a new coding and reimbursement rate for patients who are placed into OU services for these conditions. Ambulatory Patient Classification Code (APC) 0339 was designed to re- lieve some of the pressures of treating CHF patients aggressively on the front end of the process versus admitting the patients into an acute care setting. This new APC 0339 code is currently reimbursed at $408 pending that the minimal requirements for receiving this payment are met. These requirements include a stay of 8 to 24 hours, up to 48 hours, with appropriate documentation. No consideration for greater than 24 hours was made in regard to the additional OU payment. Also, most diagnostic tests that are performed during the OU stay are billable and reimbursable separately from the OU stay, as deemed medically necessary (Table 5-3).

Another "benefit" of APC 0339 for the hospital is that revisits occurring within 30 days or admissions to the hospital after an OU visit are all reimbursable. There is no restriction to the number of claims that can be submitted for a patient if billed under the APC outpatient system. Also, if a patient is admitted to an OU and then requires an inpatient hospital admission at that same point of contact, there is no "penalty." The hospital does not get the APC outpatient reimbursement but instead receives the full DRG inpatient reimbursement.

COST-EFFECTIVENESS OF THE OU

The OU provides a location for the provision of intense medical therapy and services under close observation and frequent monitoring of response to treatment. In the ADHERE data registry (a multicenter, observational database of patients discharged from the hospital with a DRG diagnosis of HF), the time to initiation of administration of certain intravenous (IV) medicines specifically directed at acute HF was 1.1 hours if the patient's

TABLE 5–3 **Comparison of Medicare Reimbursements for ADHF Financial Template**

APC 0339–CHF Inpatient	DRG 127–CHF Outpatient
Level V <8 hours $239	Avg. reimbursement $4,617
APC 0339 >8 hours $408	Mean cost $5,905
	Medicare benchmark LOS 5.3 days
UB92 Billable Reimbursable	*UB92 Billable Reimbursable*
ECG Yes Yes	ECG Yes No*
Labs Yes Yes	Labs Yes No*
ECHO Yes Yes	ECHO Yes No*
CXR Yes Yes	CXR Yes No*
IV infusion Yes Yes	IV infusion Yes No*
Drug therapy Yes Yes	Drug therapy Yes No*
	*No = bundled under the service provided
Total $XX	
Fixed cost (FC) ($ XXX)	FC ($$ XXX)
	FC varies per institution usually 3 times outpatient
Mean variable cost (VC) ($ XXX)	Mean VC ($$ XXX)
VC/FC varies per institution	All diagnostics are bundled under corresponding DRG
$XXX profit per case	($XXX) loss per case

ADHF, acute decompensated heart failure; APC, Ambulatory Patient Classification Code; CHF, congestive heart failure; CXR, chest x-ray; DRG, diagnosis-related group; ECG, electrocardiogram; ECHO, echocardiogram; IV, intravenous; LOS, length of stay.

treatment was initiated in the ED, compared with 22 hours if therapy was begun in an inpatient unit.[15] The OU has definitive protocols for both treatment and timely adjustments in treatment plans based on the clinical parameters being observed. Such a methodology leads to more intense and timely initiation of therapy. This drastic variation in timing can have remarkable differences in clinical outcomes, as well as a dramatic impact on financial implications (Figure 5–3).

Treatment of ADHF in an OU has resulted in reduced 30-day readmissions and hospitalizations and decreased LOS if a subsequent hospitalization is required.[16] The ADHERE data showed that early initiation of IV vasoactive therapy can reduce the hospital LOS from an average of 7.0 days to 4.5 days.[17] Because LOS is the greatest contributor to hospital costs for the ADHF patient, and up to 75% of ADHF cases admitted to an OU can ultimately be discharged directly from the OU, the potential impact on overall hospital utilization can be substantial.[10,18]

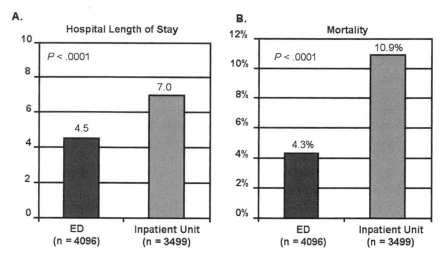

FIGURE 5–3 Effect of site initiation of therapy on length of stay and mortality. ED, emergency department. From Emerman CL. Treatment of the acute decompensation of heart failure: efficacy and pharmacoeconomics of early initiation of therapy in the emergency department. *Rev Cardiovasc Med* 2003;4(Suppl 7):S13–S20.

In an analysis of The Cleveland Clinic experience using the OU as a venue for treatment of the ADHF patient, they reported positive 90-day outcomes (Table 5–4):[19]

- Revisits were reduced by 44%
- ED observation discharges increased by 9%
- HF rehospitalizations were reduced by 36%
- Observation rehospitalizations were reduced by 39%

The authors believed this impact on outcomes was due to application of testing on presentation to the OU, patient education, and early and aggressive treatment with pharmacologic therapies.

The new APC reimbursement coding can also result in better profitability for the acute care facility. By carefully selecting appropriately risk-stratified ADHF patients and placing appropriate resources in the ED that can result in initiation of drug therapies in the 1-hour window,

TABLE 5–4 90-Day Utilization Rates in ADHF Related to OU Treatment Venue

	Before (%)	After (%)	% Change	*p* value
HF revisits	90	51	44	0.000
HF rehospitalizations	77	50	36	0.007
Death	4	1	75	0.096

ADHF, acute decompensated heart failure; HF, heart failure; OU, observation unit.

TABLE 5-5   **Utilization and Cost Differences Based on Medicare Reimbursement Type**

DRG 127 inpatient	APC 0339 outpatient
ALOS 7.0 days	ALOS 4.5 days
Avg. drug therapy Initiation = 22 hr	Avg. drug therapy Initiation = 1.1 hr
Avg. contribution margin per case = $1,288	Avg. contribution margin per case = $871
Mortality = 10.9%	Mortality = 4.3%
	Bonus reimbursement for APC 0339 = $408

ALOS, average length of stay; APC, Ambulatory Patient Classification Code; DRG, diagnosis-related group.
ALOS and mortality data based on the ADHERE registry.

hospitals can recognize a positive financial margin per case (Table 5–5). This difference in profitability comes partly from the new CMS reimbursement coding. Although the reimbursement levels for APC 0339 are smaller compared with the DRG reimbursement for a hospitalization, the operational expenses for an OU stay are also smaller. Overhead costs are generally less in the ED or outpatient units when compared with inpatient treatments because of the productivity and turnover rate of the beds. Thus, intense therapy for ADHF that results in a short stay in an OU can actually result in a profit for the hospital facility. However, the ability to show a profit in the ADHF patient still requires a redesign of the current system and attention to an early risk-stratified, protocol-driven process to be successful.

Current Medicare DRG reimbursements put extreme pressure on facilities to maintain effective treatment options available to the growing ADHF population. Facilities must explore and evaluate the advantages of using observation services that will allow the placement of traditional technologies and protocols at the point of contact with HF patients versus allowing the patients to be placed into the system only to recognize they could have been effectively identified, risk stratified, and treated more efficiently on the front end of the their presentation.

CLINICAL OUTCOMES

Process improvement initiatives appear to be the focus of government and other agencies attempting to reduce morbidity and mortality as well as increase other quality outcomes. With 550,000 new incident HF cases annually, health care delivery systems are seeing a tremendous increase in the number of patients presenting to EDs across the nation. Improved disease management and an emphasis on process are critical toward attaining improved clinical outcomes in this set of patients.

Some argue that attempts to increase quality of care are inherently more costly due to the use of more therapeutic and diagnostic interventions. However, the overall impact of high-quality care could reduce total costs by diminishing unnecessary health care utilization that results from inappropriate or inadequate care.

The Joint Commission on Accreditation of Healthcare Organizations (JCAHO) has created a set of quality performance indicators for HF.[20] These indicators include objective measurement of ejection fraction, angiotensin-converting enzyme (ACE) inhibitor treatment if tolerated, provision of complete discharge instructions, and smoking cessation counseling. In an analysis of the ADHERE registry data, only 30% of ADHF patients meet these quality requirements.[21] Although OU management has been demonstrated to reduce morbidity and a trend toward reduced mortality, further studies are needed to assess the full impact of OU care on quality measures.[22,23]

Disease management efforts for HF have demonstrated improved clinical outcomes and quality of care measures in selected populations as shown in the CMS/Premier Project launched in 2003. Clearly, third-party insurers and employers are increasingly seeking methods to merge quality care with cost reductions. Medicare has recently initiated a demonstration project to determine how disease management efforts can affect cost and quality in the senior population. Many health plans are beginning pay-for-performance programs that reward providers and facilities for providing higher quality care. Although quality appears to be the focus of such efforts, there is an underlying belief that such care will also reduce overall costs. Thus, marrying cost and quality is becoming a theme in today's health care environment.

TRANSTHEORETICAL Y-MODEL

Hospitals must merge quality and finance to create a viable plan of operation. Although this is a common concept in the business world, it has not yet been incorporated throughout the health care arena. The transtheoretical Y-model is a new approach that allows facilities to closely examine different aspects of operations within their systems.[23] It encompasses the concept of health care delivery along a continuum from the point of entry into the "system" through to discharge. This Y-model can be applied to the overall operations of these systems or to one specific disease, such as HF. By applying variations of the Y-model, in which all focus is on the end points of quality and cost, facilities can recognize ways to turn CHF from a negative contribution margin to one that breaks even or contributes favorably.

Using the transtheoretical Y-model in the health care setting can be compared with an industrial setting. Industrial facilities can examine the

ZIG-ZAG Model

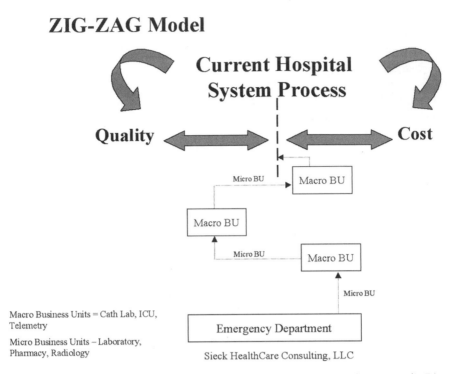

FIGURE 5-4 The zig-zag model of care. BU, business unit; ICU, intensive care unit. From Sieck S. Cost effectiveness of chest pain units. *Cardiol Clin* 2005;23(4):598.

exact route from raw material to finished product with detailed accuracy. The end product is priced to the market based on the operating costs within the process. If the manufacturing process varies greatly over time, costs of production rise and are passed on in a higher market price. To keep prices down, actions must be taken to get the variances under control. If not, the contribution margin is eroded and eventually could become negative. The objective is to keep the contribution margin at its maximum without compromising quality.

This model can be similarly applied to an ADHF patient routing through the health care delivery setting. Patients receive services within different "care units" within the acute hospital setting. These care units are analogous to the industrial setting's business units. By understanding how each care unit's operational strategies affect each subsequent care unit from point of entry to discharge, a seamless transfer of patient care in both outpatient and inpatient settings can optimize quality improvement and positive economic value. Without each care unit providing vital information to others in this holistic approach, moving patients efficiently through the system is challenged.

The current processes in health care delivery to the ADHF patient are more characteristic of a "zig-zag model" (Figure 5-4). An ADHF patient enters through the ED and receives treatments and evaluations through multiple disconnected service sectors or "care units" (known as business units in the commercial sector). These care units are represented by nursing, electrocardiogram (ECG) department, radiology department, pharmacy, laboratory, and so forth. Each of the care units is viewed and acts as a single independent business unit from the standpoint of the hospital. The outputs of these care units' activities are collated by the provider, usually once the patient has been admitted to the acute hospital bed. It is then, at the "back end" of the process, that care treatment plans are decided on. The zig-zag model is a disconnected and fragmented model.

The transtheoretical Y-model represents a different approach and provides a template to facilities on optimizing covering costs of care by placing the proper resources at the front end of the point-of-care entry. This concept begins at the point of entry and ends at discharge and marries a clinical and financial strategy that meets quality indicators while producing desirable profit margins. Beginning in the ED, this concept emphasizes an efficient, rapid assessment and action centered on a seamless integration of ancillary services, such as the laboratory, diagnostic imaging, and skilled nursing, while understanding the economic impacts on decisions made as the patient is directed through the system.

Using this template can impact quality, costs, efficiency, and clinical outcomes. This model provides a more accurate breakdown on the exact volume by *International Classification of Disease, Ninth Revision* (ICD-9) codes instead of the inpatient DRG to give a more accurate picture of the number of patients that are passing through the outpatient door within a system. With this analysis and the proper guidance, facilities can target this and other diseases more effectively. Patients who require an inpatient admission are properly admitted, and those who could be effectively treated in the outpatient setting are treated and properly released. The placement of more critical patients in the inpatient acute care setting impacts the case mix index positively because the patients are simply sicker and require more resources.

Creating a new care delivery system for the ADHF patient that is based on the transtheoretical Y-model can positively impact the contribution margins when ADHF patients are carefully identified, risk stratified, and given appropriate early treatment during the interaction (Figure 5–5). This model emphasizes a multidisciplinary team approach to align the care units that affect an ADHF patient's progress through the current system. The emphasis is on front-end compliance that sets up the pathway the patient will follow (Figure 5–6). A patient is not "arbitrarily" admitted to an inpatient bed, treated, and then discharged. A decision is made upfront on the most ideal care venue for the risk-stratified patient to be admitted to and undergo tailored treatment. It also initiates the financial pathway with identified markers throughout the patient interaction that allows facilities to know the ramifications of making random decisions versus following a protocol designed to emphasize quality while optimizing economic results. The transtheoretical Y-model places an emphasis on

Trans-theoretical Y-Model

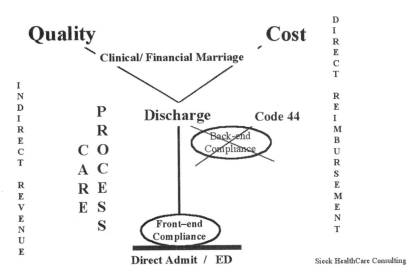

FIGURE 5–5 The transtheoretical Y-model. ED, emergency department. From Sieck S.Cost effectiveness of chest pain units. *Cardiol Clin* 2005;23(4):597.

Trans-theoretical Y-Model

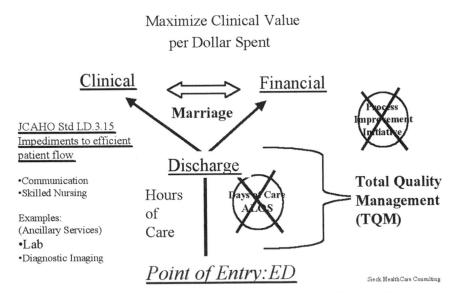

FIGURE 5–6 Use of transtheoretical Y-model to maximize cost-efficiency. ED, emergency department; JCAHO, Joint Commission on Accreditation of Healthcare Organizations. From Sieck S.Cost effectiveness of chest pain units. *Cardiol Clin* 2005;23(4):597.

Trans-theoretical Y-Model

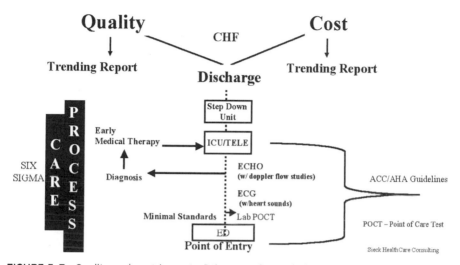

FIGURE 5–7 Quality and cost impact of the transtheoretical Y-model. ACC/AHA, American College of Cardiology/American Hospital Association CHF, congestive heart failure; ECG, electrocardiogram; ED, emergency department; ICU, intensive care unit. From Sieck S. Cost effectiveness of chest pain centers *Cardiol Clin* 2005;23(4):597.

process improvement while targeting the end points of quality and contribution margin (Figure 5–7).

This variation of the model was recently used successfully at a southern medical center for an initiative on acute coronary syndrome (ACS). Prior to the initiative the hospital had a "zig-zag" model of care. Patients entered through the ED and were admitted to the acute care bed, and laboratory tests were completed and treatment initiated several hours into the process. With initiation of the Y-model, stratification was performed and appropriate therapy initiated in the ED with point-of-care testing in a patient-centric improvement effort. The new design resulted in improvements in turnaround time for therapy, reduced LOS, enhanced patient placement in the most appropriate bed venue [e.g., critical care unit (CCU), telemetry, or clinical decision unit], and improved patient satisfaction.

Improvements demonstrated in the ACS redesign can be translated to the ADHF setting. Similar to the ACS patient, not every ADHF patient absolutely requires a CCU or OU bed. Similarly, not all ADHF patients are candidates for the OU. Point-of-entry triaging to the most appropriate care unit where an individualized treatment plan is rendered allows a facility to better merge quality care with positive financial outcomes.

CONCLUSIONS

Health care delivery systems must explore innovative strategies and health care redesign to provide cost-effective quality treatment to ADHF patients. Inconsistent and inefficient treatments contribute to poor clinical and economic outcomes. CMS is shifting patients from inpatient to outpatient services in an attempt to relieve the inpatient burden placed on hospital services while simultaneously alleviating the economic problems encountered when treating this unique class of patients. These forces create fiscal and logistic challenges for the hospital, which can ultimately impact the institution's survival.

The transtheoretical Y-model offers a solution that is focused mainly on process improvement techniques and the economic impacts these changes can have on the hospital system. The core of the model is based on merging quality and finance. Although financial aspects of care play a vital role in this model, economics cannot be considered a higher priority than clinical outcomes. The model treats these two parameters as equally important to the successful implementation of a redesigned care process for the ADHF patient population.

REFERENCES

1. Peacock WF, Albert NM. Observation unit management of heart failure. *Emerg Med Clin North Am* 2001;19:209–232.
2. Massie BM, Shah NB. Evolving trends in epidemiologic factors of heart failure: rationale for preventative strategies and comprehensive disease management. *Am Heart J* 1997;133:703–712.
3. Aghababian RV. Acutely decompensated heart failure: opportunities to improve care and outcomes in the emergency department. *Rev Cardiovasc Med* 2002;3[Suppl 4]:S3–S9.
4. Massie BM, Shah NB. Evolving trends in epidemiologic factors of heart failure: rationale for preventative strategies and comprehensive disease management. *Am Heart J* 1997;133:703–712.
5. O'Connell JB, Bristow M. Economic impact of heart failure in the United States: time for a different approach. *J Heart Lung Transplant* 1993;13:S107–S112.
6. AHA, ASA. *Heart disease and stroke statistics–2004 update.* Available at: http://www. americanheart.org/downloadable/heart/1072969766940Sstats2004Update.pdf (accessed September 13, 2004).
7. The Acute Decompensated Heart Failure National Registry (ADHERE): Opportunities to Improve Care of Patients Hospitalized with Acute Decompensated Heart Failure. Data on file January 2004.
8. Graff L, Orledge J, Radford MJ, et al. Correlation of the Agency for Health care Policy and Research congestive heart failure admission guideline with mortality: peer review organization voluntary hospital association initiative to decrease events (PROVIDE) for congestive heart failure. *Ann Emerg Med* 1999;34:429–437.
9. Emerman CL. Treatment of the acute decompensation of heart failure: efficacy and pharmacoeconomics of early initiation of therapy in the emergency department. *Rev Cardiovasc Med* 2003;4:S13–S20.
10. Peacock WF. Heart failure management in the emergency department observation unit. *Prog Cardiovasc Dis* 2004;46:465–485.

11. Aghababian RV. Acutely decompensated heart failure: opportunities to improve care and outcomes in the emergency department. *Rev Cardiovasc Med* 2002;3[Suppl 4]:S3–S9.

12. Jong P, Vowinckel E, Liv PP, et al. Prognosis and determinants of survival in patients newly hospitalized for heart failure: a population-based study. *Arch Intern Med* 2002;162:1689–1694.

13. Medicare Observation Status Reference. Volume, Issue IV, Jan 3, 2003.

14. Mace SE, Graff L, Mikhail M, et al. A national survey of observation units. *Am J Emerg Med* 2003;21:529–533.

15. Fonarow GC, for the ADHERE Scientific Advisory Committee. The Acute Decompensated Heart Failure Registry (ADHERE): opportunities to improve care of patients hospitalized with acute decompensated heart failure. *Rev Cardiovasc Med* 2003;4:S21–S30.

16. Peacock WF, Remer EE, Aponte J, et al. Effective observation unit treatment of decompensated heart failure. *Congest Heart Fail* 2002;8:68–73.

17. Peacock WF, Emerman CL, Costanzo MR, et al. Early initiation of IV vasoactive therapy improves heart failure outcome: an analysis from the ADHERE registry database. *Ann Emerg Med* 2003;42:526.

18. Peacock WF, Albert NM. Patient outcome and costs following an acute heart failure (HF) management program in an emergency department (ED) observation unit (OU) [abstract 240]. *J Heart Lung Transplant* 1999;18:92.

19. Peacock F. Management of acute decompensated heart failure in the emergency department. *J Am Coll Cardiol* 2003;4:336A.

20. www.jcaho.org

21. Fonarow GC, for the ADHERE Scientific Advisory Committee. The Acute Decompensated Heart Failure Registry (ADHERE): opportunities to improve care of patients hospitalized with acute decompensated heart failure. *Rev Cardiovasc Med* 2003;4:S21–S30.

22. Peacock WF. Acute emergency department management of heart failure. *Heart Failure Rev* 2003;8:335–338.

23. Sieck S. Cost effectiveness of chest pain units. *Cardiol Clin* 2005; 23(4):589–599, ix.

6

OBSERVATION UNIT—
TREATMENT PROTOCOLS

J. Douglas Kirk

INTRODUCTION

Although there are guidelines from various sources about the management of patients with heart failure, most pertain to chronic management.[1] Limited data are available from randomized controlled trials of acute decompensated heart failure (ADHF) patients in the emergency department (ED), much less the observation unit (OU). As a result, little consensus exists regarding their management, adding to the inconsistent care. This chapter focuses on therapeutic management, with respect to general supportive measures, pharmacologic therapy, and, most important, specific treatment protocols or algorithms that can be implemented in your institution.

GENERAL SUPPORT

The majority of patients admitted to the OU with ADHF have a chief complaint of dyspnea, and supplemental oxygen should be administered initially in essentially all patients. Pulse oximetry should be used to measure the effectiveness, with a target of maintaining an oxygen saturation of 95% or greater. This may require high-flow oxygen by facemask in some patients, whereas others may need oxygen only by nasal cannula.

Patients with severe dyspnea or hypoxia, typically seen in cases of flash pulmonary edema from severe hypertension and diastolic dysfunction (a unique syndrome more related to "hemodynamic mismatch"[2] than true "cardiac failure"), may require more aggressive airway maneuvers. In such cases, endotracheal intubation may be warranted or inevitable, but every attempt should be made to avoid intubation because of its associated morbidity in these patients. Obviously, patients this ill are not good candidates for OU care. However, the use of aggressive airway adjuncts such as noninvasive ventilation (NIV) may assist in avoiding the need for intubation while maintaining adequate oxygenation and ventilation. NIV should not be considered a substitute for intubation or, more importantly, other pharmacologic management but rather as a bridge to therapies directed at reducing filling pressures and pulmonary congestion. Further, brief periods of NIV should not exclude patients from the OU by definition, especially in patients with acute pulmonary edema from hemodynamic mismatch.

INITIAL MANAGEMENT OF ACUTE PULMONARY EDEMA

Although many patients with acute pulmonary edema are too sick for subsequent OU management, a number will turn around quickly with aggressive ED treatment, particularly those with hemodynamic mismatch. Concurrent with the previously mentioned airway maneuvers, all efforts should be directed at reducing pulmonary congestion. The most rapid improvement will be achieved with potent vasodilators such as nitroglycerin, nesiritide, or nitroprusside. Although each is quite effective, their immediate intravenous use often requires too much time to set up, a luxury these patients may not have. Initiation of sublingual nitroglycerin therapy, in doses larger than those typically used for chest pain (two to six 0.4-mg tablets or sprays) can be quite effective.[3] One can achieve significant reductions in pulmonary capillary wedge pressure and blood pressure (afterload) with an improvement in respiratory symptoms, often within minutes. Patients can then be transitioned to one of the aforementioned intravenous vasodilators and typically are reasonable candidates for the OU.

The addition of an intravenous diuretic to this strategy is common and makes some practical sense because it will result in significant diuresis and hence a drop in preload, although probably not immediately. However, a number of these patients do not suffer necessarily as much from total fluid overload as from maldistribution of fluid into the pulmonary bed. By limiting diuretic use in these patients, important deleterious effects may be avoided, confirming the primary role of vasodilators in this population (Table 6-1). Although the data are limited in the use of any of these agents in the setting of acute pulmonary edema and respiratory distress, there appears to be an immediate benefit from rapid administration of sublingual nitroglycerin with or without an intravenous loop diuretic. Further recommendations on the use of these agents cannot be made until further research elucidates the utility and safety of such an approach.

PHARMACOLOGIC THERAPY

Although general supportive measures such as maintaining adequate oxygenation are critical, the mainstay of therapy is pharmacologic. The primary goal is to decrease filling pressures. An additional important goal is improving cardiac output through a reduction in afterload or improvement in contractility. In patients with diastolic dysfunction, improving the ventricle's ability to fill with blood is key, through efforts to improve myocardial relaxation.

TABLE 6–1 **Untoward Effects of Therapeutic Agents for ADHF**

Diuretics	Vasodilators	Inotropes
Decreased renal perfusion	Tachycardia (NTG, NTP)	Increased mortality
Volume depletion	Tachyphylaxis (NTG)	Proarrhythmic
Electrolyte abnormalities (K^+, Ca^{+2}, Mg^{+2})	Neurohormonal activation (NTG, NTP)	Tachycardia
Neurohormonal activation:	Thiocyanate toxicity (NTP)	Neurohormonal activation
↑ renin-angiotensin aldosterone	Need for titration (NTG, NTP)	
↑ sympathetic nervous system	Need for invasive monitoring (NTP, ± NTG)	

ADHF, acute decompensated heart failure; NTG, nitroglycerin; NTP, nitroprusside.

Adapted from Kirk JD, Diercks DB. Acute decompensated heart failure. In: Aghababian RV, ed. *Essentials of emergency medicine.* Sudbury, MA: Jones & Bartlett, 2006: 117–124.

Diuretics

Diuretics are often first-line therapy in the OU management of patients with ADHF and as such have become a mainstay of many treatment protocols in the OU. The rationale is that patients are volume overloaded, and, although this may be true, more important than a total increase in volume is the acute elevation in filling pressures. Nonetheless, diuretics are effective in reducing preload and removing excess fluid. The loop diuretic furosemide is most commonly used, although other loop diuretics are equally effective. Suggested starting doses are 40 mg of intravenous furosemide in diuretic naive patients or an amount equivalent to the patient's total usual daily dose given intravenously. Peak diuresis should occur within 30 to 60 minutes. Repeated doses, in some instances double the initial dose, are often used in patients who fail to respond. Doses greater than 160 mg of furosemide are likely to produce as many side effects as results and should be discouraged. In patients with diuretic resistance, use of an additional diuretic that works on the proximal tubule (e.g., metolazone) may produce an effective diuresis. Caution should be exercised with excessive diuretic use. In addition to the well-described electrolyte depletion (K^+, Mg^{+2}), recent literature demonstrates that diuretics result in decreased renal perfusion and neurohormonal activation by increasing renin and norepinepherine.[4,5] The short-term gains with diuretic therapy may be offset by the decrease in renal perfusion and resultant deleterious long-term effects (Table 6–1).

Vasodilators

A minority of patients have mild exacerbations of ADHF and therapy with oxygen and loop diuretics may be sufficient, especially if their visit is due to brief periods of medical or dietary noncompliance. However, this frequently is not adequate and the addition of vasodilators becomes necessary, particularly in patients with severe hypertension and diastolic dysfunction. Most are well perfused and hence are best treated with vasodilators such as nitroglycerin, nesiritide, or nitroprusside. Some patients with mild ADHF may respond to sublingual, oral, topical, or intravenous nitrates, and several OU treatment protocols advocate this approach.[3,6] Others have promoted the use of sublingual angiotensin-converting enzyme inhibitors (ACEIs) in this setting, based largely on a small trial of 22 patients who showed symptomatic improvement after treatment with sublingual captopril.[7]

Data from ADHERE, a multicenter heart failure registry, suggest that patients treated with an intravenous vasodilator initiated in the ED versus later in the hospital or not at all had lower mortality (4.3% vs. 10.9%, unadjusted, p <0.0001) and shorter hospital lengths of stay (3 vs. 7 days, p <0.001).[8] These data generate some enthusiasm that early goal-directed therapy initiated in the ED or OU may hold promise and further study is warranted.

Despite their widespread acceptance as standard therapy, surprisingly little clinical outcome data exist for the vasodilators nitroglycerin and nitroprusside to support their use in ADHF. Physician familiarity with nitroglycerin use in patients with chest pain makes the combination of nitroglycerin and diuretics frequent first-line therapy. Nitroprusside can also be particularly useful in patients with acute pulmonary edema associated with severe hypertension but its use is uncommon. However, there are several limitations to these therapies, including the deleterious effects of neurohormonal activation and the need for titration and hemodynamic monitoring (Table 6–1). The latter two characteristics make these agents ill-suited for use in the OU. This has led to a search for better therapeutic agents, ideally ones that improve acute symptoms and hemodynamics as well as mortality. Further, ease of use is an important consideration in choosing an agent to be used in the OU.

Natriuretic Peptides

Nesiritide is the only intravenous vasodilator studied to date in the OU environment. Approved by the Food and Drug Administration in 2001, it became the first commercially available natriuretic peptide used for the treatment of ADHF. It is identical to human endogenous B-type natriuretic peptide (BNP) and serves as an antagonist to pathologic neurohormonal activation that occurs in heart failure. This feature is common among heart failure pharmacologic agents with proven mortality benefit, including ACEIs and beta-blockers. Its most important effect is the general counterbalancing of vasoconstrictive neurohormones in patients with poor cardiac output.

Nesiritide produces significant reductions in pulmonary capillary wedge pressure, right atrial pressure, and systemic venous resistance within minutes and concomitant increases in stroke volume and cardiac output.[9] In addition, it does not possess many of the untoward properties associated with diuretics, inotropes, or other vasodilators (Table 6–1). In the PRECEDENT trial, a comparison of nesiritide with dobutamine, the investigators found fewer arrhythmias and no increase in heart rate with nesiritide.[10] Data from the VMAC trial demonstrated that nesiritide decreased pulmonary capillary wedge pressure more than either nitroglycerin or standard therapy at 3 hours and more than nitroglycerin at 24 hours.[11] Dyspnea and global clinical status were improved compared with standard therapy and similar to that of nitroglycerin. In addition, nesiritide's hemodynamic effects were longer lasting, without a need for up-titration, which was frequently necessary in the nitroglycerin group to maintain adequate reduction in wedge pressure.[12] To date nesiritide is the only therapy that has been shown in randomized controlled trials of ADHF to provide significant symptomatic and hemodynamic improvement compared with placebo plus standard care.[11] However, it has not been studied in a trial prospectively designed or adequately powered to evaluate its effect on mortality, and some have questioned its safety.[13]

Nesiritide possesses several characteristics that provide convenience and ease of use: (a) no proarrhythmic effect, (b) no tachyphylaxis, and (c) no need for titration [hence not mandated for intensive care unit (ICU) use], making it quite suitable for the ED or OU population.[14]

In 237 OU patients randomized to either standard care or at least 12 hours of nesiritide therapy in the PROACTION trial,[15] the investigators report nesiritide use was associated with a substantial decrease in the sum length of stay over the ensuing month after the index OU visit (2.5 vs. 6.5 days, $p < 0.032$). Mortality and complications were uncommon and not statistically different between the two groups.

Nesiritide is typically administered as a bolus of 2 µg per kilogram followed by an infusion of 0.01 mg/kg/minute. In patients with relatively low systolic blood pressure (SBP) (90–110 mm Hg), the bolus can be reduced or eliminated altogether. If hypotension occurs, the infusion should be discontinued. It may be restarted at a lower dose when the blood pressure has stabilized, but this decision will vary on a case-by-case basis. Diuretics may be continued but typically at lower doses due to the potentiation of effects from nesiritide. ACEIs may also be used but not at the expense of curtailing the dose of nesiritide. The use of beta-blockers is not contraindicated, although their use in patients with ADHF is typically reduced or discontinued until patients are more hemodynamically stable. After therapeutic targets have been achieved, typically within 12 to 24 hours, nesiritide may be discontinued and patients should be started on proven mortality-reducing outpatient regimens (ACEI, beta-blocker, aldosterone antagonist) with appropriate adjustments in dosing based on clinical status.

Inotropes

The use of inotropes has essentially no role in the OU management of patients with ADHF. Patients exhibiting clear signs of decreased perfusion or overt cardiogenic shock should be managed in an ICU with appropriate hemodynamic monitoring, and thus further discussion here is not warranted.

MANAGEMENT ALGORITHMS IN THE OBSERVATION UNIT

Appropriate management of ADHF in the ED and/or OU is challenging. Conclusive evidence identifying suitable patients who clearly benefit from a particular therapy is lacking, as are specific guidelines to drive management. It does appear, however, that patient risk stratification[16] and initiation of aggressive treatment in the ED[8] may limit potentially irreversible myocardial toxicity, especially in those with moderate to severe ADHF. The algorithm depicted in Figure 6–1 attempts to provide some guidance for the diagnostic and prognostic evaluation of the suspected ADHF patient, in addition to recommendations for therapeutic strategies and disposition decisions.[17] For the purposes of this chapter's focus on OU care, sections pertaining to the potentially life-threatening complications of respiratory failure or cardiogenic shock are not discussed in detail.

Using typical historical, physical examination, and diagnostic test features, a clinical profile is defined, identifying patients in whom pulmonary congestion predominates the clinical presentation versus those with more of an element of hypoperfusion. A minority of patients will have mild exacerbations of ADHF, and the mainstay of therapy for them may be intravenous diuretics, particularly if they have been noncompliant with diet or medications. Topical or sublingual nitrates may be warranted if moderate hypertension (SBP 140- 160 mm Hg) is present or a history of diastolic dysfunction exists.

The majority of ADHF visits are of moderate severity and often characterized by significant hypertension. An abrupt increase in blood pressure may precipitate acute pulmonary edema, especially in patients with diastolic dysfunction. This presentation is more related to hemodynamic mismatch. Accordingly, the clinical target is blood pressure control with early, aggressive vasodilation, more so than diuresis. This is particularly true when pulmonary congestion is related to fluid maldistribution more than an increase in total fluid volume. Preliminary data suggest these patients should be aggressively treated with intravenous vasodilators early in the ED course,[8] and a substantial number may be appropriate for OU management.[15] The ideal choice of a specific vasodilator in these cases can be difficult. Nitroglycerin and loop diuretics are effective in symptomatically improving these patients but are associated with neurohormonal activation and several limitations to their ED or OU use (Table 6–1). From a practical standpoint, the most important limitation is the need for titration and admission to an ICU. In many institutions, this renders these agents ineffectual because their use would not be permitted in the OU setting. If for no other reason, the use of nesiritide and its characteristic ease of use may play a significant role here. Using the guidelines to estimate severity from Figure 6–1, the majority of patients classified as moderate risk and those at low risk can all be managed in an OU.

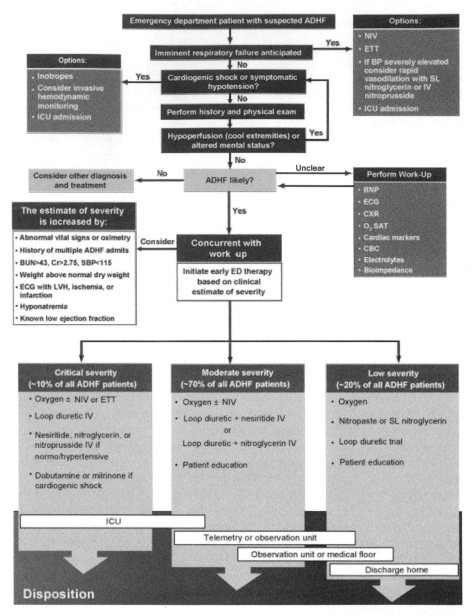

FIGURE 6–1 Algorithm for the early stabilization of acute decompensated heart failure in the emergency department. ADHF, acute decompensated heart failure; BNP, B-type natriuretic peptide; BUN, blood urea nitrogen; CBC, complete blood count; Cr, creatinine; CXR, chest radiograph; ECG, electrocardiogram; ETT, endotracheal tube; ICU, intensive care unit; LVH, left ventricular hypertrophy; NIV, noninvasive ventilation; O_2SAT, oxygen saturation; prn, as needed; SBP, systolic blood pressure; SL, sublingual. (Adapted from Peacock WF, Allegra J, Ander D, et al. Management of acutely decompensated heart failure in the emergency department. *CHF* 2003;9[Suppl 1]:3–18.)

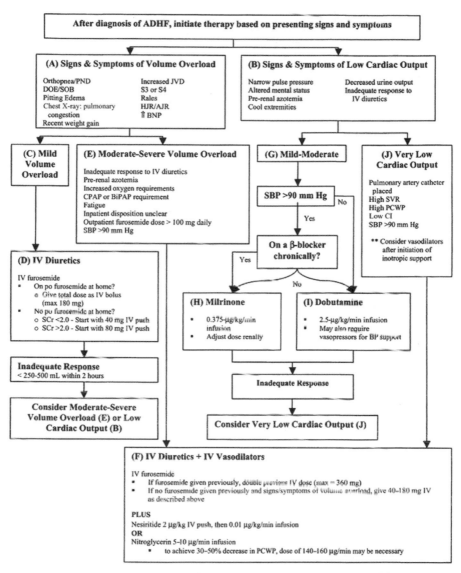

FIGURE 6–2 Acute decompensated heart failure (ADHF) treatment algorithm. AJR, abdominal jugular reflex; BiPAP, bilevel positive airway pressure; BNP, B-natriuretic peptide; CI, cardiac index; CPAP, continuous positive airway pressure; DOE, dyspnea on exertion; HJR, hepatojugular reflex; JVD, jugular venous distention; PCWP, pulmonary capillary wedge pressure; PND, paroxysmal nocturnal dyspnea; SBP, systolic blood pressure; SCr, serum creatinine; SOB, shortness of breath; SVR, systemic vascular resistance. (Adapted from DiDomenico RJ, Park HY, Southworth MR, et al. Guidelines for acute decompensated heart failure treatment. *Ann Pharmacother* 2004;38:649–660, with permission.)

Another algorithm with more patient-specific treatment recommendations for management of ADHF in the OU was reported by DiDomenico et al.[18] and is described in Figure 6–2. The timeline for key elements of these guidelines is depicted in Figure 6–3 and provides

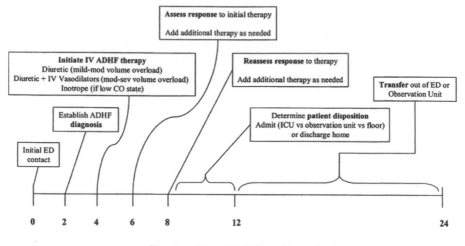

FIGURE 6–3 Timeline for the management of acute decompensated heart failure (ADHF) in the emergency department/observation unit. CO, cardiac output; ED, emergency department; ICU, intensive care unit; mod-sev, moderate to severe. (Adapted from DiDomenico RJ, Park HY, Southworth MR, et al. Guidelines for acute decompensated heart failure treatment. *Ann Pharmacother* 2004;38:649–660.)

clinicians with specific clinical targets that should be achieved during the OU stay. The authors felt strongly that the diagnosis of ADHF should be established within 2 hours after presentation to the ED. Intravenous therapy should be initiated within 2 hours of establishing the diagnosis, and within 2 hours of initiating intravenous therapy the patient's response should be assessed and additional therapy added as necessary. Over the following 6 to 8 hours, reassessment of the patient's response should continue, and after 12 hours of observation, disposition should be determined (i.e., hospital admission or discharge home). Transfer out of the OU should then proceed within 24 hours of the initial OU contact.

In this strategy, treatment of ADHF is generally based on the presence or absence of volume overload and an assessment of the patient's cardiac output. On the left side of Figure 6–2 (boxes A, C, D, E, and F) treatment recommendations are given for patients with ADHF experiencing signs and symptoms of volume overload, manifested by pulmonary congestion. One of the limitations of this algorithm is grouping all patients with pulmonary congestion together, regardless of the etiology. There is no consideration of the patient with hemodynamic mismatch and acute pulmonary edema, whose primary therapy should be control of blood pressure with intravenous vasodilators. Nonetheless, it is quite helpful with general management principles. The right side of the algorithm provides treatment recommendations for patients with low cardiac output.

In most OUs these patients are excluded, and therefore little discussion of this component of the algorithm is warranted.

The major emphasis of this protocol is managing volume overload, which is further divided into mild and moderate-severe groups. Patients with mild volume overload (Figure 6–2, box C) are treated with intravenous diuretic therapy, typically loop diuretics (Figure 6–2, box D). Dosages in patients previously taking diuretics are guided by the total home daily dose, given as an intravenous bolus. Therapy for patients not taking oral diuretics at home is based on renal function, although clinicians should exercise caution with diuretic therapy in such patients to avoid further worsening of renal function. Success of diuretic therapy is driven by urine output goals and recommendations for repeat diuretic dosing are described in the algorithm. Again, caution should be exercised with extremely high doses of loop diuretics. In addition to the prerenal azotemia, electrolyte abnormalities, particularly hypokalemia and hypomagnesemia, are common and should be recognized and treated quickly. A management strategy for electrolyte disturbances in this setting is included in the accompanying standing orders (Figure 6–4).

The authors recognize that patients with more severe volume overload, which typically includes those with hemodynamic mismatch and resultant acute pulmonary edema, are likely to have an inadequate response to intravenous diuretic therapy alone. In these patients, the initial pharmacologic regimen should be more aggressive and include both an intravenous diuretic and a parenteral vasodilator (Figure 6–2, box F). Intravenous nitroglycerin or nesiritide should be used to produce a more rapid response and more effectively relieve the signs and symptoms of congestion in these patients. No specific recommendations are provided as to which vasodilator should be used. However, untoward effects of conventional vasodilators (Table 6–1) and ease of use characteristics associated with nesiritide therapy should be considered when choosing the optimal agent to be used in the OU. Further, the suggested starting dose of nitroglycerin (5–10 µg per minute) noted in Figure 6–2, box F should be considerably higher.

Corresponding physician order sets for ADHF management in the OU have been developed and are presented in Figure 6–4. These are a vital part of any OU management algorithm and are typically necessary to standardize the evaluation and treatment of ADHF patients. These orders are for sample purposes only and should be modified accordingly to accommodate institutional variations in practice. Again, the inclusion of orders for inotropic therapy in this example is typically not permitted in the majority of observation units.

Similar algorithms have also been published by other groups and warrant mention here to provide alternatives and to highlight important differences in OU management strategies. The Midwest Heart Specialists Heart Failure Program produced an algorithm for the early goal-directed therapy of ADHF patients (Figure 6–5).[19] Several key decision points are

Congestive Heart Failure Order Set
For Acute Decompensated Congestive Heart Failure Patients
Emergency Department Order Sheet

Date   Time   Primary Diagnosis: Acute Decompensated Congestive Heart Failure
Secondary Diagnosis: _____
Vital signs q4h and as directed by medications (see individual medications)

❑ Labs: Basic metabolic panel, calcium, magnesium, phosphorus, CBC, PT/INR, PTT, BNP, CK, CK-MB, Troponin, O₂ saturation
❑ Digoxin level (if outpatient medication)
❑ Patient Weight: _____
❑ Ins and Outs
❑ 12 Lead ECG
❑ AP and lateral chest x-ray
❑ Foley catheter prn heavy diuresis
❑ Diet: <2.4g Na, low fat
❑ Fluid restriction: 1800 mL/24h; if Na <131 mg/dL, restrict fluid to 1500 mL/24h

Intravenous Furosemide
❑ If furosemide naïve, furosemide 40 mg IVP x 1 dose
❑ If on furosemide as outpatient
   Total daily dose as IV _____ mg: maximum 180 mg
   • Goal: >500 mL urine output within 2 hours for normal renal function
     >250 mL urine output within 2 hours if renal insufficiency
   • If goal urine output not met within 2 hours, double the furosemide dose to a maximum of 360 mg IV
   • Monitor symptom relief, vital signs, BUN, SCr, electrolytes

Nesiritide
❑ 2 µg IV push followed by 0.01 µg/kg/min IV infusion
❑ If symptomatic hypotention during infusion, discontinue nesiritide
   • Monitor symptom relief, vital signs q15m × 1 hour, then q30min × 1 hour, then q4h, urine output, electrolytes, BUN, SCr, magnesium, calcium, phosphorus
❑ If poor symptom relief or diuretic response ≥3 hours after nesiritide therapy initiation AND SBP ≥90 mm Hg, may consider titration of nesiritide
   • Nesiritide 1 µg/kg IVP and increase infusion by 0.005 µg/kg/min
   • May increase infusion rate q1h after first dosage, increase to a maximum dose of 0.03 µg/kg/min

Nitroglycerin 50 mg/250 mL
❑ 5 µg/min IV infusion; titrate dose q5min by 10–20 µg/min to achieve symptom relief
   • Monitor symptom relief, vital signs q15min until stable dose, then q30min × 1 hour, then q4h ECG, urine output

FIGURE 6–4 Physician order set for the initial management of acute decompensated heart failure in the emergency department/observation unit. AP, anterior/posterior; BNP, B-natriuretic peptide; BUN, blood urea nitrogen; CBC, complete blood cell count; CK, creatine kinase; CK-MB, creatine kinase MB isoenzyme; ECG, electrocardiogram; INR, international normalized ratio; IVP, intravenous push; PT, prothrombin time; PTT, partial thromboplastin time; SBP, systolic blood pressure; SCr, serum creatinine; Clcr, creatinine clearance. (Adapted from DiDomenico RJ, Park HY, Southworth MR, et al. Guidelines for acute decompensated heart failure treatment. *Ann Pharmacother* 2004;38: 649–660.) *(continued)*

emphasized: (a) early and accurate diagnosis of ADHF with clinical variables and BNP testing; (b) identification of those ADHF patients with shock, followed by prompt admission; (c) treatment of the ADHF patient with renal insufficiency with vasoactive medication; and (d) frequent

Dobutamine 500 mg/250 mL
❑ 2.5 µg/kg/min IV infusion and titrate dose every 5 minutes to desired response to a maximum dose
     of 20 µg/kg/min
      • Monitor symptom relief, vital signs q15min until stable dose, then q30min × 1 hour, then
        q4h; ECG; urine output

Milrinone 20 mg/100 mL
❑ 0.375 µg/kg/min
      • Monitor symptom relief, vital signs q15min until stable dose, then q30min × 1 hour, then
        q4h; ECG; urine output

❑ Digoxin   _____
                     Dose   Route   Frequency

❑ Lisinopril PO _____
                     Dose   Frequency

❑ Losartan PO _____
                     Dose   Frequency

❑ Metoprolol PO _____
                     Dose   Frequency

❑ Spironolactone PO _____
                     Dose   Frequency

Electrolyte Replacement
❑ Potassium

level (mEq/L)	IV dose (over 1 h)	PO dose	When to recheck potassium
3.7–3.9	20 mEq	40 mEq	12 hours or next morning
3.4–3.6	20 mEq × 2 doses	40 mEq × 2 doses	6 hours or next morning
3.0–3.3	20 mEq × 4 doses	40 mEq × 3 doses	4 hours after last dose
<3.0	20 mEq × 6 doses	Give IV only	1 hour after last dose

      • If Clcr <30 mL/min, reduce dose by 50%

❑ Magnesium

level (mEq/L)	IV dose	PO dose (Mg oxide)	When to recheck magnesiun
1.9	Give PO only	140 mg	Next morning
1.3–1.8	1 g MgSO₄ for every 0.1 below 1.9 (max 6 g)	Give IV only	Next morning
<1.3	8 g MgSO₄	Give IV only	6 hours after last dose or next morning

      • MgSO$_4$ 1–2 g, infuse over 1 hour
      • MgSO$_4$ 3–6 g, infuse ≤2 g/hour

_____   _____
Physician Signature   Date

FIGURE 6–4 *(continued)*

re-evaluation of the ED/OU treated patient to identify early treatment fail-
ures, followed by prompt institution of vasoactive therapy in these patients. In
many instances, treatment recommendations are similar to those proposed by
DiDomenico et al.[18] However, important differences include distinguishing
patients with renal insufficiency and instituting early intravenous nesiritide

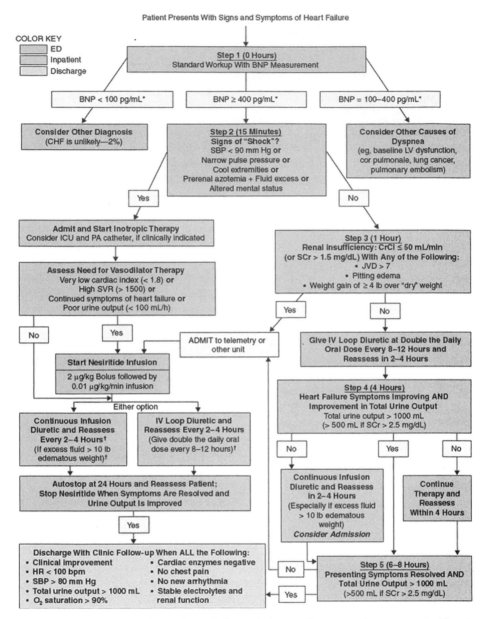

FIGURE 6–5 Algorithm for early goal-directed therapy for acute decompensated heart failure. ED, emergency department; BNP, B-type natriuretic peptide; CHF, congestive heart failure; ICU, intensive care unit; PA, pulmonary artery; SVR, systemic vascular resistance; HR, heart rate; SBP, systolic blood pressure; LV, left ventricular; CrCl, creatinine clearance; SCr, serum creatinine; JVD, jugular venous distention. *Clinical decisions should not be based solely on BNP level. BNP levels shown are for the Triage (Biosite) assay. †Consider decreasing dose of diuretic by 50% if receiving nesiritide. (Adapted from Saltzberg MT. Beneficial effects of early initiation of vasoactive agents in patients with acute decompensated heart failure. *Rev Cardiovasc Med* 2004;5[Suppl 4]:S17–S27.)

plus continuous infusion of a loop diuretic or bolus loop diuretic. Nitroglycerin therapy is not included in this approach. Also, patients without renal insufficiency are treated with bolus loop diuretic monotherapy and reassessed every 2 to 4 hours. Those who fail to improve and/or do not achieve urine output targets are started on continuous infusion loop diuretics. Failure to improve by 6 to 8 hours prompts additional therapy with intravenous nesiritide. Similar to the aforementioned algorithm,[18] patients with acute pulmonary edema due to hemodynamic mismatch are not distinguished with respect to initial therapy with intravenous vasodilators.

Using the Midwest heart algorithm, an analysis of data before and after implementation provided insight into the potential impact of such an approach.[19] Hospital and telemetry unit length of stay was significantly reduced among patients with concomitant renal insufficiency and those requiring intravenous vasoactive therapy. Vasoactive use increased after algorithm utilization but still was seen in only one third of all hospitalized ADHF patients. In patients with renal insufficiency, the treatment algorithm resulted in a doubling of nesiritide use when compared with similar patients for whom the algorithm was not used. Nesiritide use as an overall percentage of vasoactive therapy (50%) was unchanged, and only 15% of all ADHF patients who were subsequently admitted had been treated with nesiritide. Despite the increased use of nesiritide, overall drug costs and costs associated with vasoactive therapy were actually reduced, suggesting that an early goal-directed approach can be implemented in a cost-effective manner while simultaneously improving outcomes.

CONCLUSIONS

Evidence-based guidelines for the management of ADHF patients in the ED and OU are lacking. Although treatment protocols and management algorithms appear vital to the success of any OU strategy, they are currently based largely on anecdotal experience or, at best, data from small trials. Cornerstones of these algorithms are appropriate patient risk stratification and recognition of those primarily with pulmonary congestion versus those with cardiogenic shock. Further delineation based on (a) severity of volume overload, (b) associated renal insufficiency, or (c) hemodynamic mismatch as an etiology appears to aid with management decisions. Unfortunately, there is no consensus among authors regarding an overall approach. Systematic use of therapeutic agents (intravenous diuretics and vasodilators) with a priori defined clinical targets is a must. Further, data seem to support the early use of vasodilators in the ED or OU,[8] and nesiritide in particular appears well suited for the OU setting.[15] Additional recommendations await publication of institutional experience with algorithms such as those presented here.

REFERENCES

1. Hunt SA, Baker DW, Chin MH, et al. ACC/AHA guidelines for the evaluation and management of chronic heart failure in the adult: executive summary. A report of the American College of Cardiology/American Heart Association Task Force on Practice Guidelines (Committee to revise the 1995 Guidelines for the Evaluation and Management of Heart Failure). *J Am Coll Cardiol* 2001;38:2101–2113.

2. Gheorghiade M, Zannad F, Sopko G, et al. for The International Working Group on Acute Heart Failure Syndrome. Acute heart failure syndrome: current state and framework for future research. *Circulation* 2005;112(25):3958–3968.

3. Bussmann W, Schupp D. Effect of sublingual nitroglycerin in emergency treatment of severe pulmonary edema. *Am J Cardiol* 1978;41:931–936.

4. Gottlieb SS, Brater DC, Thomas I, et al. BG9719 (CVT-124), an A1 adenosine receptor antagonist, protects against the decline in renal function observed with diuretic therapy. *Circulation* 2002;105:1348–1353.

5. Brewster UC, Setaro JF, Perazella MA. The renin-angiotensin-aldosterone system: cardiorenal effects and implications for renal and cardiovascular disease states. *Am J Med Sci* 2003;326:15–24.

6. Cotter G, Metzkor E, Kaluski E, et al. Randomised trial of high-dose isosorbide dinitrate plus low-dose furosemide versus high-dose furosemide plus low-dose isosorbide dinitrate in severe pulmonary oedema. *Lancet* 1998;351:389–393.

7. Hamilton RJ, Carter WA, Gallagher EJ. Rapid improvement of acute pulmonary edema with sublingual captopril. *Acad Emerg Med* 1996;3:205–212.

8. Peacock WF, Emerman CL, Costanzo MR, et al. Early initiation of intravenous vasoactive therapy improves heart failure outcomes: an analysis from the ADHERE registry database. *Ann Emerg Med* 2003;42:S26.

9. Mills RM, LeJemtel TH, Horton DP, et al. On behalf of the Natrecor Study Group. Sustained hemodynamic effects of an infusion of nesiritide (human B-type natriuretic peptide) in heart failure: a randomized, double-blind, placebo-controlled clinical trial. *J Am Coll Cardiol* 1999;34:155.

10. Burger AJ, Horton DP, LeJemtel T, et al. Effect of nesiritide (B-type natriuretic peptide) and dobutamine on ventricular arrhythmias in the treatment of patients with acutely decompensated congestive heart failure: the PRECEDENT study. *Am Heart J* 2002;144:1102–1108.

11. Publication Committee for the VMAC Investigators. Intravenous nesiritide vs nitroglycerin for treatment of decompensated congestive heart failure: a randomized controlled trial. *JAMA* 2002;287:1531–1540.

12. Elkayam U, Akhter MW, Singh H, et al. Comparison of effects on left ventricular filling pressure of intravenous nesiritide and high-dose nitroglycerin in patients with decompensated heart failure. *Am J Cardiol* 2004;93:237–240.

13. Sackner-Bernstein JD, Kowalski M, Fox M. Short-term risk of death after treatment with nesiritide for decompensated heart failure. A pooled analysis of randomized controlled trials. *JAMA* 2005;293:1900–1905.

14. Fonarow GC, ADHERE Scientific Advisory Committee. The Acute Decompensated Heart Failure National Registry (ADHERE): opportunities to improve care of patients hospitalized with acute decompensated heart failure. *Rev Cardiovasc Med* 2003;4[Suppl 7]: S21–S30.

15. Peacock WF, Holland R, Gyarmathy R, et al. Observation unit treatment of heart failure with nesiritide: results from the PROACTION trial. *J Emerg Med* 2005;29(3):243–252.

16. Fonarow GC, Adams KF Jr, Abraham WT, et al, for the ADHERE Scientific Advisory Committee, Study Group, and Investigators. Risk stratification for in-hospital mortality in acutely decompensated heart failure: classification and regression tree analysis. *JAMA* 2005;293:572–580.

17. Peacock WF, Allegra J, Ander D, et al. Management of acutely decompensated heart failure in the emergency department. *CHF* 2003;9[Suppl 1]:3–18.

18. DiDomenico RJ, Park HY, Southworth MR, et al. Guidelines for acute decompensated heart failure treatment. *Ann Pharmacother* 2004;38:649–660.

19. Saltzberg MT. Beneficial effects of early initiation of vasoactive agents in patients with acute decompensated heart failure. *Rev Cardiovasc Med* 2004;5[Suppl 4]:S17–S27.

7

DRUGS THAT SHOULD NOT BE USED IN THE OBSERVATION UNIT MANAGEMENT OF HEART FAILURE: THE ADVERSE EFFECTS OF SELECTED DRUGS

Harischandra B. Karunaratne,
Arti N. Bhavsar, and Nicole Rosenke

It is estimated that approximately 1 million patients are discharged from the hospital annually with a diagnosis of chronic heart failure (HF). As the population ages, the prevalence of HF will increase significantly. The number of patients admitted to the hospital with HF continues to grow at an unprecedented rate. Eighty percent of men and 70% of women younger than 65 years diagnosed with HF will die within 8 years. Long-term survival following the diagnosis of HF has been found to be better in women than in men. However, less than 15% of women diagnosed with HF survive more than 8 to 12 years. The mortality rate in this cohort is high, with one in five patients dying within 1 year.[1] Recognizing the devastating effects of various medications on the exacerbation of HF, this discussion focuses on best practices in the drug therapy management of patients with HF.

One third of all HF patients admitted to the hospital are readmitted for the same condition within 90 days. Analysis of the factors leading to this high readmission rate shows many preventable causes. Nearly 50% of readmissions are due to noncompliance either with a salt-restricted diet or with prescribed drug therapy. Sixteen percent of all hospital readmissions due to exacerbation of HF are associated with the use of inappropriate medications.[2]

These findings have led to the development of disease management programs based on clinical guidelines and standardized protocols designed to improve and optimize outcomes of both the in-patient and outpatient treatment of HF. These approaches use trained nurse clinicians and advanced nurse practitioners focusing on patient education during the in-patient stay. These programs also provide follow-up supervision through telephone contact and outpatient monitoring. Close attention is paid to weight gain, adherence to a salt-free diet, appropriate adjustment of diuretic dosage, and potassium supplements. Moreover, the continuation of evidence-based care with angiotensin-converting enzyme (ACE) inhibitors, angiotensin receptor blockers (ARB), and beta-blockers is maintained.

Many patients with HF are elderly with multiple comorbid conditions and require long-term follow-up. The concomitant use of medications that have the potential to precipitate or exacerbate HF or to produce life-threatening arrhythmias must be closely monitored. Often, these drugs may have been prescribed by another physician for the treatment of a comorbid chronic condition such as diabetes mellitus or may be inadvertently consumed by the patient for the temporary relief of some type of ailment, for example, an over-the-counter nonsteroidal anti-inflammatory drug (NSAID) for arthritic pain.

The "2005 Guidelines for Diagnosis and Management of Chronic Heart Failure in the Adult"[3] lists three classes of drugs that can exacerbate HF and that should be avoided in these patients. These include antiarrhythmic agents, calcium channel blockers, and NSAIDs.

Table 7–1 is a comprehensive list of medications that have the potential to precipitate or worsen HF. An extensive review of the literature has been conducted. Two excellent reports, by Amabile and Spencer[4] and Feenstra et al.,[5] have eloquently addressed the issue of medications that exacerbate HF.

In this discussion, agents traditionally used in the treatment of acute or chronic HF that may have potentially serious side effects have been excluded. Consideration of certain other medications is beyond the scope of this discussion, including chemotherapeutic agents such as the anthracyclines, cyclophosphamide, trastuzumab (Herceptin), and paclitaxel and the immunomodulating agents interferon-alpha and -gamma and interleukin-2. In addition, the adverse cardiovascular effects of anesthetic agents and the effects of recreational drugs are not addressed.

Drug-induced exacerbation of HF may occur for varying reasons. It may take place in patients with impaired left ventricular (LV) function due to increased cardiac afterload, as a result of increased systemic vascular resistance from vasoconstriction. It may also result from a rise in preload due to fluid retention and volume expansion and the depression of cardiac contractility caused by negative inotropy of drugs. However, other factors may also play an important role in producing adverse outcomes in HF. Some of these mechanisms are summarized in Table 7–2.

ANTI-INFLAMMATORY AGENTS

Anti-inflammatory agents are the most widely used medications that exacerbate HF. These include corticosteroids, NSAIDs, and selective cyclooxygenase 2 inhibitors (coxibs).

TABLE 7–1 **Drugs that Precipitate or Exacerbate Chronic Heart Failure**

- Anti-inflammatory medications
- Cardiovascular medications
- Diabetic medications
- Neurologic and psychiatric medications
  Amphetamines
  Carbamazepine
  Clozapine
  Ergot alkaloids
  Pergolide
  Tricyclic antidepressants
- Chemotherapeutic agents
  Anthracyclines
  Cyclophosphamide
  Paclitaxel
  Herceptin
- Antifungal medications
  Itraconazole
- Anesthetic agents
  Halogenated volatile anesthetics
  Intravenous barbiturate anesthetics
- Herbal medications
  Ephedra
  Licorice
- Recreational drugs
- Immunomodulating agents
  Interferon-alpha, -gamma
  Interleukin-2
- Miscellaneous medications
  Drugs with high sodium content
  Beta 2 agonists

Corticosteroids

Corticosteroids are frequently used in clinical practice for the treatment of a broad array of common diseases such as asthma, chronic obstructive pulmonary disease (COPD), and multiple allergic conditions and as immunosuppressive agents in organ transplantation. Their use for these purposes in HF patients has not been specifically addressed. These drugs

TABLE 7–2 **Mechanisms by Which Drugs May Exacerbate Chronic Heart Failure**

Mechanism
• Direct cardiotoxicity
• Negative inotropy
• Arrhythmogenicity
QT prolongation
Sympathoadrenal stimulation
• Fluid and sodium retention
• Renal insufficiency
• Electrolyte imbalance
• Drug interactions
• Mediated via CYP3A4 metabolism in liver

often cause sodium and fluid retention, plasma volume expansion, and a loss of hypertensive control.

Elevation of blood pressure by corticosteroids appears to be mediated by a decrease in the nitric oxide–mediated vasodilatation and increased responsiveness to vasoconstrictors.[6] Because of the likelihood of exacerbation of HF, patients using these drugs should be closely monitored for weight gain, diuresis, and blood pressure control. The dose and duration of a course of these drugs should be minimized, and the requirement for continuation of steroids should be frequently assessed. The use of drugs with minimal mineralocorticoid activity is also helpful.[4]

Nonsteroidal Anti-Inflammatory Drugs

NSAIDs act primarily through their ability to inhibit prostaglandin synthesis, by blocking cyclo-oxygenase. Renal prostaglandins play an important role in maintaining kidney perfusion in patients with HF. The use of NSAIDs, even in a single dose, may significantly reduce glomerular filtration rate, leading to sodium and water retention and plasma volume expansion.[7] These agents also reduce the effectiveness of diuretics in HF.

Elderly patients who have New York Heart Association (NYHA) Class III and IV HF and have been stabilized with diuretics have an increased rate of hospitalization for worsening symptoms when given NSAIDs (other than aspirin).[8] The multiple NSAIDs currently available do not appear to have any difference in their ability to exacerbate HF. Hospitalization rate for HF exacerbation appears to be highest early after the initiation of these agents.

The use of NSAIDs in patients with HF should always be avoided. Although elderly patients on large doses of loop diuretics are at greatest risk, younger individuals are likely to show exacerbation with these drugs. If the use of these agents cannot be avoided, close monitoring for the deterioration of renal function, weight gain, dyspnea, and edema is of critical importance.

The use of acetylsalicylic acid (ASA) along with ACE inhibitors has been the focus of much research discussion.[8] Results from retrospective studies appear to justify the use of ASA and ACE inhibitors when there is a clear indication for the use of ASA, as in patients with ischemic dilated cardiomyopathy. However, others have claimed that because ASA inhibits cyclo-oxygenase and prostaglandin synthesis, it may blunt the beneficial effects of ACE inhibitors. From the currently available data, the potential likelihood of reduced ACE inhibitor effectiveness does not appear to overcome the known beneficial effects of ASA, primarily in patients with ischemic heart disease.

Cyclo-Oxygenase II Inhibitors

Coxibs were originally developed to reduce an adverse effect profile in relation to reduced gastrointestinal bleeding.[9] Coxibs selectively block cyclo-oxygenase 2, which accumulates at sites of inflammation. It was originally postulated that they would not interfere with prostaglandin production in the gastric mucosa or renal parenchyma or at sites of platelet aggregation. However, currently available data leave unresolved the issue that these drugs may be prothrombotic. Cox 2 appears to be present in the human kidney and its inhibition leads to fluid and sodium retention. Based on these findings, coxibs do not appear to have any advantage over the conventional NSAIDs with reference to fluid retention and the aggravation of HF.

Table 7–3 summarizes the influence of anti-inflammatory medications on the exacerbation of HF. The type of medication, mode of adverse reaction, and appropriate recommendations are presented.

CARDIOVASCULAR MEDICATIONS

Certain cardiovascular medications are known to have adverse effects in HF. These include antiarrhythmic drugs as well as some antihypertensive agents and are listed in Table 7–4.

Antiarrhythmics

The management of ventricular arrhythmias in patients with HF has evolved over the last decade. Empiric therapy with antiarrhythmic drugs has a limited role in the management of patients with ventricular arrhythmia and LV dysfunction. It is generally limited to the use of one agent, amiodarone, in asymptomatic patients with nonsustained ventricular tachycardia (VT) who are otherwise not candidates for electrophysiologic study and/or device therapy. Vaughn-Williams Class I and the Class III agents sotalol and ibutilide should not be used to treat ventricular arrhythmias in patients with LV dysfunction because of their proarrhythmic and negative inotropic activity. Electrophysiology (EP) study–guided

TABLE 7-3 Anti-Inflammatory Medications That Exacerbate Chronic Heart Failure

Medication	Mode of Adverse Reaction	Recommendations
Corticosteroids	• Sodium and fluid retention • Loss of hypertensive control	• Monitor for decompensation • Minimize dose and duration • Choose agent with least mineralocorticoid activity • Periodically assess for necessity

NSAIDs	• Sodium and water retention
	• Blunted diuretic response
	• Increased systemic vascular resistance
		• Avoid non-ASA NSAIDs in HF
		• Cox II inhibitors offer no advantage to patients with heart failure over conventional NSAIDs
		• If NSAID use cannot be avoided
		  1. Monitor weight
		  2. Assess dyspnea

Cox II inhibitors	• Fluid retention
	• Exacerbation of hypertension
	• Impairment of renal function
	• Possible thrombolic events
		• Avoid in HF
		• If it cannot be avoided
		  1. Monitor weight gain
		  2. Assess dyspnea
		  3. Watch blood pressure, renal function

ASA, acetylsalicylic acid; HF, heart failure; NSAIDs, nonsteroidal anti-inflammatory drugs.

TABLE 7–4 Cardiovascular Medications That May Exacerbate Chronic Heart Failure

- Antiarrhythmic agents
  1. Vaughn-Williams Class Ia, Ic agents
     a. Procainamide
     b. Quinidine
     c. Disopyramide
     d. Flecainide
  2. Some Class III agents
     a. Sotalol
     b. Ibutilide
- Antihypertensive agents
  1. Alpha-adrenergic blockers
  2. Calcium channel blockers
  3. Minoxidil
- Drugs used in the treatment of peripheral vascular disease
  1. Cilostazol

antiarrhythmic and/or device therapy is now the standard of care in this cohort of patients.[3]

Drug therapy in patients with atrial fibrillation (AF) complicating HF represents a more difficult problem. Approximately 20% to 30% of patients with AF also have a history of HF. The age-adjusted odds ratio for AF in patients with HF is 6:8. In the Stroke Prevention in Atrial Fibrillation (SPAF) study, a post hoc analysis showed an increased incidence of cardiac death in patients with HF and AF who were treated with antiarrhythmic agents.[10] Although sometimes used for AF, Class I antiarrhythmic agents, including quinidine, procainamide, disopyramide, flecainide, and propafenone, are negatively inotropic to varying degrees and have proarrhythmic potential. They should not be used in the treatment of AF associated with HF and/or LV dysfunction.

The Class III agent sotalol, a mixture of the D and L isomers, is often used to maintain sinus rhythm once AF patients have been converted to normal sinus rhythm.[11] Its use in patients with LV dysfunction and concomitant HF is not recommended because of reports of a higher likelihood of the occurrence of polymorphic VT (torsades de pointes). A clinical trial using only the D-isomer of sotalol (D-sotalol), a drug that has only Class III arrhythmic properties and no significant beta-blocking effect, showed an increased mortality risk in patients with ejection fraction less than 40%.[12]

Ibutilide, a Class III antiarrhythmic agent, is often used as an initial intravenous infusion over a 10-minute period for restoration of sinus rhythm in patients with AF. In one placebo-controlled double-blind randomized clinical trial, Ellenbogen et al.[13] reported that 6 of 197 patients (3.0%) developed VT. All 6 patients had LV systolic dysfunction. Based on these findings, ibutilide should not be used for arrhythmia conversion in patients presenting with both AF and HF. Two other Class III agents, amiodarone and dofetilide, are the only antiarrhythmic agents that can be administered safely to maintain sinus rhythm in patients with AF and LV systolic dysfunction.

Antihypertensive Drugs

The "2005 Guidelines for Diagnosis and Management of Chronic Heart Failure in the Adult"[3] classifies HF into four stages: A, B, C, and D. Stage A HF comprises patients at high risk but without structural heart disease and symptoms. One of the most important subgroups in Stage A includes patients with hypertension (HTN). Antihypertensive therapy in these patients prevents worsening the progression of HF from Stage A to asymptomatic LV dysfunction.

ALPHA-ADRENERGIC BLOCKERS. Recent studies have suggested that certain drugs that are effective antihypertensive agents and can be safe in patients with Stage A HF may actually worsen or aggravate the condition when used in Stage B and beyond. The alpha-adrenergic blocking agent prazosin is an effective vasodilator and antihypertensive. However, it was found to be no better than placebo in the V-heft I study.[14] In the ALLHAT study, the alpha-blocker doxazosin was associated with an increased risk of developing HF.[15] As a result, this drug was withdrawn from the study prematurely.

In the recently published "2005 Guidelines for Diagnosis and Management of Chronic Heart Failure in the Adult"[3] update, alpha-blockers, although not specifically contraindicated, are not among the antihypertensive medications listed as useful in the treatment of various stages of HF. They do still fill a role in the treatment of symptomatic benign prostatic hypertrophy. The use of alpha-blockers in patients with HF for such purposes should be discouraged and minimized, because adverse effects such as orthostatic hypotension may frequently occur in these patients.

CALCIUM CHANNEL BLOCKERS. The nondihydropyridine calcium channel blockers verapamil and diltiazem have both negative chronotropic and negative inotropic effects. They have been demonstrated to be associated with deteriorating HF when used in patients with LV dysfunction. Although diltiazem is less negatively inotropic and chronotropic than verapamil, the use of both of these agents as antihypertensive therapy in patients with LV dysfunction and HF is not recommended.

Diltiazem is often used in combination with beta-blockers and digoxin when a rate control strategy is used in patients with AF. When patients with LV dysfunction are managed by rate control, the use of beta-blockers and digoxin is preferred to diltiazem alone or in combination.

Admittedly, in certain patients the benefit of effective rate control with combination therapy (beta-blockers, digoxin) may be great enough to permit the use of diltiazem along with these drugs, even in patients with LV dysfunction. Limiting diltiazem to the smallest effective dose is recommended in such situations. Alternative rate control strategies such as atrioventricular nodal ablation and pacing should also be considered.

Dihydropyridine calcium channel blockers do not have significant negative chronotropy. The two long-acting dihydropyridine calcium channel blockers amlodipine and felodipine have not shown any adverse outcomes in patients with HF. In a study conducted with amlodipine, a group of patients with nonischemic dilated cardiomyopathy did show modest benefits.[16]

On the other hand, the calcium channel blockers nifedipine, nisoldipine, and isradipine have demonstrated clinical deterioration and increased hospitalization in HF and are therefore contraindicated in these patients. They appear to produce this effect by their negative inotropic activity and detrimental activation of the renin-angiotensin axis and sympathoadrenal system. Consequently, if calcium channel blockers must be used, the preferred choice is amlodipine or felodipine.

MINOXIDIL. Minoxidil is a potent arterial vasodilator. It causes a significant drop in blood pressure for hypertensive patients through its reduction of systemic vascular resistance by direct smooth muscle relaxation. The drug causes extensive fluid retention and edema formation. Increasing doses of loop diuretics may be required in NYHA Class III or IV HF patients. It is best to avoid the use of this agent for this group of patients.

Cardiovascular Agents Used in the Treatment of Peripheral Vascular Disease

CILASTOZOL. Cilastazol (Pletal) is an agent that is used for treatment of intermittent claudication in patients with peripheral vascular disease. It is a phosphodiesterase III inhibitor and has been shown to increase heart rate, the frequency of premature ventricular contractions, and nonsustained VT. Adverse outcomes have been reported in patients with HF who have been treated with other oral phosphodiesterase inhibitors, such as oral amrinone or milrinone. Therefore, the use of cilostazol in patients with HF is not recommended.

DIABETIC MEDICATIONS

Metformin

Metformin is a biguanide used in the treatment of type II diabetes, either alone or in combination with other oral agents. It acts by decreasing hepatic glucose production. It is most useful in the treatment of overweight diabetics. A small number of patients taking the drug, 0.03 cases per 1,000 patients, develop lactic acidosis, which increases the risk of mortality by

50%. Metformin is renally eliminated and hence the risk of lactic acidosis is highest in patients with renal insufficiency. In a study of 47 patients with metformin-related lactic acidosis, 38% had HF.[17] Consequently, metformin should not be used in patients with NYHA Class III or IV HF and diabetes.

Thiazolidinediones

As many as 12% of patients with type II diabetes have HF. The thiazolidinediones (TZDs) rosiglitazone and pioglitazone are used alone or in combination to treat type II diabetes. An estimated 2% to 5% of patients on monotherapy with these drugs and 5% to 15% of patients receiving concomitant insulin therapy will develop peripheral edema and weight gain. A recent study showed that these agents increase intravascular volume by 6% to 7%.[18] Development of HF and pulmonary edema as early as 3 days and as late as 13 months after initiating treatment with TZD has been described.[19] The mechanism of fluid retention is currently unknown. However, it responds better to drug withdrawal than to diuretic therapy.

No direct adverse effect of TZD on cardiac function has been reported. Moreover, fluid retention appears to be independent of cardiac function. There is also a considerable body of knowledge that suggests that TZDs may have significant positive effects on cardiac function, including reduced vascular resistance, improved cardiac metabolism, and coronary vasodilation. If TZDs are used in patients with diabetes, careful monitoring for new or aggravated HF is essential. This group of drugs should be avoided in NYHA Class III or IV HF.

Table 7–5 summarizes the influence of diabetes medications on the exacerbation of HF. The type of medication, mode of adverse reaction, and appropriate recommendations are presented.

NEUROLOGIC AND PSYCHIATRIC MEDICATIONS

Amphetamines

Amphetamines have been used to treat narcolepsy. However, more recently, they have been used in children and adults for the treatment of attention deficit hyperactivity disorder. These agents release norepinephrine, which stimulates both alpha and beta receptors, thereby increasing blood pressure and heart rate. Because sympathetic activation can promote arrhythmia in patients with HF, these drugs should be avoided in patients with HF.

Tricyclic Antidepressants

Traditionally, these agents have been used to treat depression and insomnia. However, with the advent of selective serotonin reuptake inhibitors, they are now more frequently used to treat migraine and neuropathic pain. These

TABLE 7–5 **Diabetes Medications That Exacerbate Chronic Heart Failure**

Medication	Mode of Adverse Reaction	Recommendations
Metformin	• Rarely leads to lactic acidosis (30 per million patients) • In one study, 38% of patients with lactic acidosis had HF • The drug is renally eliminated and hence levels rise within liver causing increased lactate levels	• Avoid use in Class III/IV HF • Patients with recurrent hospitalization for HF • Avoid if serum creatinine >1.5 mg/dL (males) or >1.4 mg/dL (females)
Thiazolidinediones (TZDs)	• Edema and weight gain–volume expansion–exacerbation of HF • Concomitant insulin use with TZD, increases HF risk	• Avoid use with Class III/IV HF • May continue to use in selected patients (if other agents are inadequate or unacceptable) • Monitor weight gain, edema if HF symptoms worsen

HF, heart failure.

medications have a known proarrhythmic potential and have always been used with caution in patients with heart disease. Anecdotal case reports have also indicated a potential but rare risk of developing cardiomyopathy and HF.[5] The use of these agents should be avoided in patients with HF.

Table 7–6 summarizes the influence of neurologic and psychiatric medications on the exacerbation of HF. The type of medication, mode of adverse reaction, and appropriate recommendations are presented.

HERBAL MEDICATIONS

Herbal medications are widely used in this country. It is estimated that in the United States 3% of English-speaking adults and a much larger number of non–English-speaking adults take herbal medications. Despite the widespread use of herbal remedies, very little is known about the safety, quality control, or efficacy of these agents.

The use of digitalis preparations, derived from the foxglove plant to treat HF, date back more than 200 years. Adverse effects resulting from toxicity with this drug, including ventricular arrhythmias and heart block, are well recognized. However, owing to the lack of published data, little is known about the adverse effects of other herbal remedies on HF.

TABLE 7–6 Neurologic and Psychiatric Medications That Exacerbate Chronic Heart Failure

Medication	Mode of Adverse Reaction	Recommendations

Amphetamines	• Release norepinephrine into central nervous system
	  1) Agonist activity results in elevated blood pressure
	  2) Escalated doses result in tachycardia
	• Increase sympathetic activity; detrimental in HF patients because they are more susceptible to arrhythmias
		• Contraindicated in patients with advanced atherosclerosis, symptomatic CVD, HTN (HF patients often have at least one of these)
		• Consider alternative therapy for narcolepsy/ADHD/hyperactivity

Carbamazepine	• Negative inotropic and chronotropic activity
	• Suppression of sinus nodal automaticity and atrioventricular conduction can induce:
	  1) Bradycardic effect
	  2) LV dysfunction
		• Avoid in HF patients (particularly elderly and those with underlying heart disease)
		• If necessary, keep within tight therapeutic range

Clozapine	• Unknown association between cardiomyopathies and clozapine use • Supporting evidence 1) Australian Clozapine Registry reports cardiomyopathies to be five times higher in clozapine users[4]	• Avoid in HF patients • If last resort, frequent assessment of ventricular function

(continued)

TABLE 7–6 Neurologic and Psychiatric Medications That Exacerbate Chronic Heart Failure (continued)

Medication	Mode of Adverse Reaction	Recommendations

Ergot alkaloids	• Valvular abnormalities that complicate HF[4]
	• Ergotamine
	  1) High norepinephrine levels
	  2) Cardiac remodeling
	• Methysergide
	  1) High 5HT levels and activity
	  2) Valvular fibrosis
		• Avoid use, if possible, in HF patients
		• If used, monitor for new-onset murmurs, bruits and friction rubs
		• Long-term prognosis—**avoid**

Pergolide	• Dopamine receptor antagonist • Excess 5HT levels resulting in valvular fibrosis similar to the ergot alkaloids[4]	• Avoid use, if possible • Baseline ECG and cardiovascular exam • Closely observe patients for new onset of HF symptoms 1. Discontinue at first sign/symptom

Tricyclic antidepressants (TCAs)	• Class Ia antiarrhythmic activity (proarrhythmic potential)
	• Case reports indicate:
	  1) HF symptoms were directly related to duration of therapy and plasma concentration
	  2) HF symptoms resolved on discontinuing TCAs
		• SSRIs
		• Neuropathic pain/insomnia
		  1. Consider other agents, specifically for elderly patients

ADHD, attention deficit hyperactivity disorder; ECG, electrocardiogram; CVD, cardiovascular disease; HF, heart failure; SSRIs, selective serotonin reuptake inhibitors.

Ephedra

Ephedra or Ma Huang has been used in Chinese medicine for thousands of years. Ephedra contains several alkaloids, including ephedrine and pseudoephedrine, all of which are sympathomimetic and directly or indirectly increase heart rate, cardiac output, blood pressure, and peripheral vascular resistance.[20] Ephedra has been used in the treatment of asthma and in narcolepsy to stimulate the central nervous system as well as for depressive states. Recently, ephedra has been marketed for weight loss and performance enhancement in a wide range of over-the-counter products. In February 2004, the U.S. Food and Drug Administration banned the use of ephedra-containing products citing, among others, its ability to increase mortality due to HF and sudden death in patients with chronic HF and coronary artery disease.[21]

Licorice

Licorice is derived from the roots of a plant, *Glycyrrhiza glabra,* and is often used as a candy and in the treatment of dyspeptic symptoms. The active agent is similar to carbenoxalonesodium and causes fluid retention, hypokalemia, and HTN and exacerbates HF.[10] It also appears to enhance aldosterone activity. It should not be used in patients with HF.

MISCELLANEOUS MEDICATIONS

In patients with HF, attention must be directed to the high sodium content of some medications. For example, the excessive use of sodium-containing antacids may exacerbate HF. In conditions such as bacterial endocarditis, large doses of intravenous antibiotics with a high sodium content may also precipitate HF. Clearly, every effort must be made to treat HF patients with agents that have a reduced sodium content.

SUMMARY

The medical management of patients presenting with HF represents a significant challenge. Hospitalizations are continuing to increase at an unprecedented rate in this cohort of patients. Many of these hospitalizations can be attributed to the exacerbation of preexisting HF. Dietary indiscretion, noncompliance with prescribed drug therapy, and the use of inappropriate medications are frequently found to be major factors responsible for HF patient cardiac decompensation.

Several drugs that exacerbate HF are often used in the treatment of comorbid conditions commonly found in an aging population. This includes arthritis, diabetes, HTN, and AF. An awareness of the possible adverse reactions of drugs used to treat these common comorbid conditions is essential in making rational therapeutic decisions for HF patients.

REFERENCES

1. American Heart Association. *Heart disease and stroke statistics–2005 update.* Dallas, TX: American Heart Association, 2005.

2. Aghababian RV. Acutely decompensated heart failure: opportunities to improve care and outcomes in the emergency department. *Rev Cardiovasc Med* 2002;3[Suppl 4]: S3–9.

3. Hunt SA, American College of Cardiology, American Heart Association Task Force on Practice Guidelines (Writing Committee to update the 2001 Guidelines for the Evaluation and Management of Heart Failure). ACC/AHA 2005 Guideline update for the diagnosis and management of chronic heart failure in the adult: A report of the American College of Cardiology/American Heart Association Task Force on Practice Guidelines (Writing Committee to Update the 2001 Guidelines for the Evaluation and Management of Heart Failure). *J Am Coll Cardiol* 2005;46:e1–e82.

4. Amabile CM, Spencer AP. Keeping your patient with heart failure safe: a review of potentially dangerous medications. *Arch Intern Med* 2004;164:709–720.

5. Feenstra J, Grobbee DE, Remme WJ, Stricker BH. Drug-induced heart failure. *J Am Coll Cardiol* 1999;33:1152–1162.

6. Worth JA, Schyvens CG, Zhang Y, et al. The nitric oxide system in glucocorticoid-induced hypertension. *J Hypertens* 2002;20:1035–1043.

7. Feenstra J, Heerdingk ER, Grobbee DE, Stricker BHCh. Association of nonsteroidal anti-inflammatory drugs with first occurrence of heart failure: The Rotterdam Study. *Arch Intern Med* 2002;162:265–270.

8. Page J, Henry D. Consumption of NSAIDs and the development of congestive heart failure in elderly patients: an underrecognized public health problem. *Arch Intern Med* 2000;160:777–784.

9. Whelton A, Fort JG, Puma JA, et al. Cyclooxygenase-2–specific inhibitors and cardiorenal function: a randomized, controlled trial of celecoxib and rofecoxib in older hypertensive osteoarthritis patients. *Am J Ther* 2001;8:85–95.

10. Flaker GC, Blackshear JL, McBride R, et al. Antiarrhythmic drug therapy and cardiac mortality in atrial fibrillation. The Stroke Prevention in Atrial Fibrillation Investigators. *J Am Coll Cardiol* 1992;20:527–532.

11. Antonaccio MJ, Gomoll A. Pharmacologic basis of the antiarrhythmic and hemodynamic effects of sotalol. *Am J Cardiol* 1993;72:27A–37A.

12. Waldo AL, Camm AJ, deRuyter H, et al. Effect of d-sotalol on mortality in patients with left ventricular dysfunction after recent and remote myocardial infarction: The SWORD Investigators. Survival With Oral d-Sotalol. *Lancet* 1996;348:7–12.

13. Ellenbogen KA, Stambler BS, Wood MA, et al. Efficacy of intravenous ibutilide for rapid termination of atrial fibrillation and atrial flutter: a dose-response study. *J Am Coll Cardiol* 1996;28:130–136.

14. Cohn JN, Archibald DG, Ziesche S. Effect of vasodilator therapy on mortality in chronic congestive heart failure. Results of a Veterans Administration Cooperative Study. *N Engl J Med* 1986;314:1547–1552.

15. The ALLHAT Officers and Coordinators for the ALLHAT Collaborative Research Group. Major cardiovascular events in hypertensive patients randomized to doxazosin vs chlorthalidone: the Antihypertensive and Lipid-Lowering Treatment to Prevent Heart Attack Trial (ALLHAT). *JAMA* 2000;283:1967–1975.

16. Packer M, O'Connor CM, Ghali JK, et al. Effects of amlodipine on morbidity and mortality in severe chronic heart failure: Prospective Randomized Amlodipine Survival Evaluation Study Group. *N Engl J Med* 1996;335:1107–1114.

17. Misbin RI. The phantom of lactic acidosis due to metformin in patients with diabetes. *Diabetes Care* 2004;27:1791–1793.

18. Kennedy FP. Do thiazolidinediones cause congestive heart failure? *Mayo Clin Proc* 2003;78:1076–1077.

19. Kermani A, Garg A. Thiazolidinedione-associated congestive heart failure and pulmonary edema. *Mayo.Clin Proc* 2003;78:1088–1091.

20. Dhar R, Stout CW, Link MS, et al. Cardiovascular toxicities of performance-enhancing substances in sports. *Mayo Clin Proc* 2005;80:1305–1315.

21. *FDA News P04-17*. (February 6, 2004). FDA issues regulation prohibiting sale of dietary supplements containing ephedrine alkaloids and reiterates its advice that consumers stop using these products. Available at http://www.fda.gov/bbs/topics/NEWS/2004/NEW01021.html (accessed October 13, 2005).

8

PERFORMANCE MEASUREMENT, STAFFING, AND FACILITIES REQUIREMENTS FOR OBSERVATION UNIT HEART FAILURE MANAGEMENT

Nancy M. Albert

When planning to open a heart failure (HF) management program in a chest pain center (also known as a short stay or observation unit), there are behind-the-scenes aspects to consider that promote optimal patient outcomes. Even though emergency care quality indicators are not specific to HF management, a substantive HF program should meet performance standards deemed important to inpatient and ambulatory HF care. Thus, the purpose of this chapter is to discuss performance measurement specific to HF care. Staffing and facilities requirements are discussed because they provide the structure and process aspects of a quality HF program that advances performance scores to improve patient quality of life, decrease morbidity, and reduce the quantity and length of hospitalization episodes.

PERFORMANCE MANAGEMENT

No specific HF performance measures exist for a HF management program in a short stay unit setting. Performance measures were developed for hospitalized and ambulatory patients with HF by national organizations (Table 8–1) to improve the quality and consistency of care that hospitalized patients receive and to provide expectations of quality ambulatory care for programs that wish to be certified as a HF disease management program.

The Joint Commission on Accreditation of Healthcare Organizations (JCAHO) developed the HF Core Measure Set in 2002 as one of four initial priority focus areas for hospital core measure development. Measuring the processes and outcomes of hospital care for patients with HF increases health care provider awareness that HF is a highly prevalent condition, uses more Medicare dollars for diagnosis and treatment than any other diagnosis, and is a common Medicare diagnosis-related group, reflecting

(*Text continues on page 91.*)

TABLE 8–1 **Performance Measures in Heart Failure**

Measure 0 = Outpatient I = Inpatient	Source	Description	Rationale
Patient education–predischarge [I] or during an ambulatory visit [O] including drug doses and frequency [O]	ACC/AHA; JCAHO	Documentation that patients received written instructions or educational materials that includes content on activity level, diet, medication administration, follow-up appointment, weight monitoring, and understanding symptoms and what to do if they worsen	Nonadherence to HF therapies and self-care is often a cause of rehospitalization. Knowledge of HF prognosis and care expectations is a prerequisite to self-care and therapy adherence.[22,23] An effective management strategy is close attention and follow-up of prescribed medications to proactively recognize potential interactions and minimize adverse effects.[22]
Assessment of left ventricular systolic function–I and O	ACC/AHA; JCAHO	Documentation that left ventricular function was previously assessed, assessed in hospital, or there are plans to assess postdischarge–I	Other assessment methods, in combination (history, physical exam, chest x-ray, and ECG), are unreliable for distinguishing between left ventricular systolic dysfunction, preserved left ventricular function, or a noncardiac etiology.[22]
Use of ACEI or ARB in patients with left ventricular systolic dysfunction–I and O	ACC/AHA–ACEI or ARB; JCAHO–ACEI	Documentation of prescribing an ACEI or ARB in patients with systolic HF (prior to discharge–I) when there are no contraindications documented	Multiple large, randomized studies of ACEIs in patients with systolic HF showed that it alleviated symptoms, improved clinical status, enhanced quality of life, and reduced the risk of death and hospitalization.[22]

(continued)

TABLE 8–1 **Performance Measures in Heart Failure** (continued)

Measure 0 = Outpatient I = Inpatient	Source	Description	Rationale
Use of beta-blocker in patients with left ventricular systolic dysfunction–I and O	OPTIMIZE-HF researchers	Documentation of prescribing a beta-blocker with known benefit in patients with systolic HF (prior to discharge–I) when there are no contraindications documented	Multiple large, randomized studies of beta-blockade in patients with systolic HF showed that it alleviated symptoms, improved clinical status, enhanced quality of life, and reduced the risk of death and hospitalization.[22]
Smoking cessation counseling and advice–I and O	ACC/AHA; JCAHO	In adults with a history of smoking cigarettes (defined as smoking in the last 1 year prior to admission), documentation of smoking cessation counseling or advice (prior to discharge–I)	Smoking has cardiotoxic effects.[22] Many deaths in the United States are attributed to a smoking-related illness. Additionally, up to one half of patients with cardiovascular disease begin smoking again within 12 months of their diagnosis.[24]
Use of warfarin in patients with HF and atrial fibrillation–I and O	ACC/AHA	In patients with chronic or recurrent (persistent, permanent, or paroxysmal) atrial fibrillation, documentation of prescribing warfarin (prior to discharge–I) when there are no contraindications documented	Stasis of blood in the fibrillating atria may predispose patients to systemic or pulmonary emboli. Prevention of thromboembolic events is an essential element of HF treatment.[25]

TABLE 8–1 **Performance Measures in Heart Failure** (continued)

Measure 0 = Outpatient I = Inpatient	Source	Description	Rationale
Initial laboratory tests–O	ACC/AHA	Initial laboratory evaluation to include urinalysis and serum testing for complete blood count, basic serum electrolytes (including serum creatinine), calcium, magnesium, blood lipids, glycohemoglobin, and thyroid stimulating hormone	Hyper- and hypothyroidism can be a primary or contributing cause of HF. Other laboratory tests can reveal illnesses or disorders that exacerbate or cause HF.[22]
Weight measurement–O	ACC/AHA; JCAHO	Obtain a weight at each visit; assess for weight change, reflecting a change in volume status	Provides clues about volume status that is essential in determining sodium status (excess or deficiencies) that may precipitate the need for diuretic therapy, self-care knowledge/adherence in low-sodium diet and fluid management (in volume overload) or changes in drug therapies (hypovolemia).[22]
Blood pressure measurement–O	ACC/AHA; JCAHO	Obtain a blood pressure at each visit	Elevated systolic and diastolic blood pressure is a risk for development of HF,[22] and high blood pressure in HF portends worse outcomes (due to worsened left ventricular remodeling).[22]

(continued)

TABLE 8–1 **Performance Measures in Heart Failure** (continued)

Measure 0 = Outpatient I = Inpatient	Source	Description	Rationale
Assessment of clinical symptoms of (excess) volume overload–O	ACC/AHA	Assess for dyspnea, fatigue, and orthopnea at each visit	Same rationale as weight monitoring.
Assessment of clinical signs of (excess) volume overload–O	ACC/AHA	Assess for peripheral edema, rales, hepatomegaly, ascites, S_3 or S_4 gallop, and elevated jugular venous pressure at each visit	Same rationale as weight monitoring.
Assessment of activity level–O	ACC/AHA	Assess level of activity using a standardized scale or tool at every visit to evaluate the impact of HF on activity level (functional status)	Questions about level of activity might provide greater insight into functional limitations than asking about symptoms experienced because many patients curtail activities when symptoms interfere.[22]
Assessment of return for emergency care or admission to the hospital–O	JCAHO[a]	90-day return for emergency care or hospitalization for HF after the index emergency care discharge for HF	Hospital discharges for HF rose 157% from 1979 to 2002.[24] Risk of hospitalization, return emergency care visit, and death within 3 months of discharge from emergency care for HF was high: 61% of patients, in a single-center study.[26]
Screened for or given influenza vaccination–O	JCAHO[a]	The number of patients with HF who are screened for or given an influenza vaccination	In patients with HF, influenza can lead to a complex HF decompensation and death.

TABLE 8–1 **Performance Measures in Heart Failure** (continued)

Measure 0 = Outpatient I = Inpatient	Source	Description	Rationale
			Influenza is a serious concern for patients with HF because there is a high risk for complications, hospitalization, and worse outcomes. A vaccination may prevent needless illness and hospitalization.[5]
Screened for or given pneumococcal vaccination– O	JCAHO[a]	The number of patients with HF who are screened for or given a pneumococcal vaccination	Same rationale as influenza vaccine; high rate of death from a preventable bacterial disease. Pneumococcal infection can increase HF exacerbation, hospitalization, morbidity, and mortality.[3]

ACC, American College of Cardiology; ACEI, angiotensin-converting enzyme inhibitor; AHA, American Heart Association; ARB, angiotensin receptor blocker; ECG, electrocardiography; HF, heart failure; JCAHO, Joint Commission on Accreditation of Healthcare Organizations.
[a]These standardized HF measurements are exclusive to JCAHO as part of their disease-specific care certification. They have been posted for public comment (now closed to comments) but have not been finalized.

frequent hospitalizations.[1] The four standardized core measures set for hospitalized patients are discharge instructions, assessment of left ventricular function, use of an angiotensin-converting enzyme inhibitor (ACEI) in patients with left ventricular dysfunction, and smoking cessation advice and counseling. These measures provide a starting point for addressing key aspects of HF care.

In addition to the four JCAHO core measures, researchers from the Organized Program to Initiate Lifesaving Treatment in Hospitalized patients with Heart Failure (OPTIMIZE-HF), a registry and performance improvement program for patients hospitalized with HF, found that discharge use of a beta-blocker was safe and well tolerated, improved treatment rates, and was associated with lower risk of mortality.[2] Researchers concluded that the data were compelling enough to warrant adding discharge use of a beta-blocker as an HF performance measure.[2]

The American College of Cardiology (ACC) and American Heart Association (AHA) developed performance measures for chronic HF. In addition to the four JCAHO core predischarge hospital measurements, a fifth measure was applied: use of an anticoagulant in patients with atrial fibrillation. In these performance measures, use of an ACEI was expanded to include angiotensin receptor blockade as an equivalent drug class.[3]

Although the JCAHO and ACC/AHA HF core measures and OPTIMIZE-HF beta-blocker measure were developed for patients hospitalized with HF, they should be applied in a short stay HF management program. These six core measures are easy to assess and implement when facility planning includes the resources necessary for patient education, left ventricular function assessment, and ordering of core HF medications. Of note, in a study of JCAHO core measures applied at a two-campus university hospital health care system, availability of standardized order forms, computer discharge instructions, and education materials did not lead to improvement in core measures scores; however, a dedicated nurse practitioner implementing resources led to rapid and sustained improvements.[4] Clearly, having a champion to develop, implement, and continually monitor the quality of care patients receive is an asset to HF management program success. In a short stay unit setting that does not use a dedicated advance practice nurse, nursing and physician personnel who make up the team must understand the importance of consistent application of core performance measures to achieve outcomes consistent with long-term goals of HF management: to cause reversal or prevent progression of left ventricular remodeling.

Performance measures have been developed for ambulatory HF management programs by ACC/AHA[3] and JCAHO.[5] Table 8.1 includes 15 performance measures, many of which are essential to both inpatient and outpatient HF care. There is not 100% agreement in stated performance measures by ACC/AHA and JCAHO; however, each measure is an essential element in improving specific clinical HF care. Because a short stay unit visit is uniquely different from an in-patient hospital stay or a chronic ambulatory visit, the 15 ACC/AHA and JCAHO performance measure profiles should be applied in a short stay HF management program but require some revision to fully apply. In Table 8–2, four measures from Table 8–1 were modified for use in a short stay HF management program. Rationale for the suggested changes is provided in Table 8–2.

Thus far, performance measures have been described with rationale for use. Placing words on paper is much easier than developing and implementing systems that promote reaching predetermined benchmarks for each performance standard. The next sections discuss staffing and facilities requirements that will help programs meet performance measures.

TABLE 8–2 **Modified Performance Measurements for a Short Stay HF Management Program**

Measure	Description	Rationale for Modification
Assessment of left ventricular systolic function	Documentation that left ventricular function was previously assessed or assessed during short-stay visit. If previous assessment reported diastolic dysfunction and was <1 year ago, repeat assessment during short stay visit.	Chest x-ray and ECG are insufficient in determining specific cardiac abnormalities. The treatment plan, including medication and intervention therapies, is based on left ventricular function and ejection fraction percent.[22] A change in clinical status due to previous therapies provides useful information about next steps in therapy.[22]
Use of ACEI or ARB in patients with left ventricular systolic dysfunction	Same as Table 8–1; however, "use" includes ensuring the right dose and using with a diuretic agent if current status includes volume overload. A short stay visit provides an opportunity to titrate ACEI or ARB therapy based on clinical status, comorbid conditions, and current dose.	Because of favorable effects on survival, treatment should not be delayed unless contraindications or adverse effects exist. Higher dosage is more likely to reduce hospitalizations but not symptoms or mortality. Goal: achieve prespecified doses used in large, clinical trials (target dosage).[22]
Use of beta blocker in patients with left ventricular systolic dysfunction	Same as Table 8–1; however, "use" includes ensuring the right drug, the right dose, and concurrent use of diuretic therapy if fluid overload (to maintain sodium and fluid balance and prevent exacerbation of fluid overload). A short stay visit provides an opportunity to ensure beta-blocker therapy is appropriate based on chronic HF guidelines.	Beta-blockers do not have a class effect. Three agents (carvedilol, metoprolol succinate, and bisoprolol) are safe and effective for use in systolic HF in patients who are clinically stable.[22] Initiate at low dose and uptitrate in gradual increments to prespecified target dose (based on dosages used in large clinical trials).[22] Patients are more likely to remain on beta-blocker therapy after discharge when it is initiated prior to hospital discharge.[2,27]

(continued)

TABLE 8–2   **Modified Performance Measurements for a Short Stay HF Management Program** (continued)

Measure	Description	Rationale for Modification
Initial laboratory tests	Same as Table 8–1 (initial evaluation) plus the following at *each encounter*: complete blood count, basic serum electrolytes (including serum creatinine), and BNP level.	In patients with acute dyspnea treated in an emergency care department, rapid BNP measurement improved evaluation and treatment and reduced costs of treatment and length of time to discharge.[28]
Other measures from Table 8–1	Same as Table 8–1	Same as Table 8–1

ACEI, angiotensin-converting enzyme inhibitor; AHA, American Heart Association; ARB, angiotensin receptor blocker; BNP, B-type natriuretic peptide; ECG, electrocardiography; HF, heart failure.

STAFFING

To determine staffing needs in a short stay unit HF management program, a review of the literature included studies of patients treated in an emergency care short stay unit, in a hospital, and in an outpatient setting. Very few groups prospectively studied the safety, cost, and outcomes of HF management in an emergency department short stay unit, and there were no randomized trials that compared outcomes of an emergency care–based short stay unit HF management program with a hospital admission.[6,7] Of the published emergency care, hospital, and outpatient management studies, no information on staffing was reported in study designs except to describe caregiver type in programs as combination physician/nurse, advance practice nurse, multidisciplinary (i.e., home care nursing or pharmacist involvement), or physician led.

Because staffing was not a theme found in the literature, studies were reviewed of HF management by caregiver. There were many reports of differences in outcomes by physician caregiver type. Cardiologist participation improved guideline adherence,[8] reduced the risk of composite death and cardiovascular hospitalization in outpatients[8] and in newly hospitalized patients,[9] increased use of diagnostic testing, and improved clinical outcomes in hospitalized patients.[10] In a self-report study design between primary care physicians and cardiologists, cardiologists were more likely to conform to published guidelines for chronic HF than were internists and family practitioners,[11] and when cardiologists were compared with HF specialty cardiologists, HF specialists were more likely to conform to chronic HF guidelines than cardiologists.[12] In a survey of family physicians and cardiologists, family physicians had less understanding of chronic HF pathophysiology and how treatment differed according to underlying disease processes. Family physicians were more likely to overestimate the risk of ACEI and warfarin use, resulting in underprescribing of therapies.[13] In a retrospective cohort study conducted with national databases, cardiology care and cardiology care mixed with general practitioner care was associated with improved survival compared with general practitioner care alone.[14] In a qualitative study of HF in primary care, perceived obstacles to evidence-based diagnosis and management were lack of time and expertise.[15] Physicians reported having difficulty with diagnosis (due to nonspecific symptoms) and not having confidence in initiating an ACEI. Moreover, many general practitioners were unaware of the impact of ACEIs on morbidity and mortality.[15]

The literature provides evidence that there is a gap between science and practice by physician caregiver type. There was no literature that compared HF care by emergency care physicians, general practitioners, cardiologists, or HF specialty cardiologists; however, emergency care physicians may be similar to general practitioners in that they must have a broad range of knowledge to care for a broad patient population. Their focus in training is more likely to be on emergent and acute situations rather than conditions that fall into the category of chronic care. Thus, emergency care physicians who oversee HF management programs in a short stay unit may require additional knowledge and training to provide HF care that is consistent with adherence to national HF guidelines.

No research literature was found on nurse staffing requirements for a short-stay HF management program. There were articles in the literature of "specialized" HF or cardiovascular nurses providing care that led to improved outcomes over usual care. However, in most cases, the setting was a HF disease management program led by HF specialty cardiologists. Advanced practice nurses (nurse practitioners or clinical nurse specialists) provided some aspects of care but did not provide independent care.[16,17] In other reports, nurses worked collaboratively with physiotherapists, social workers, and case managers.[18,19] Thus, encouragement and support must be provided to all caregivers involved in clinical management. Nurse caregivers, who are likely to be responsible for patient education, must be properly educated before they can teach others. In a study of nursing knowledge of HF patient education principles, nurses who regularly cared for patients with HF had a mean score of 75% correct on a survey of statements applicable to patient education principles. Scores were highest for HF specialty nurses and lowest for cardiology floor nurses.[20] Therefore, emergency care nurses responsible for patient education may also require additional education.

Short stay unit nurses are responsible for patient assessment, drug delivery and monitoring, review of laboratory results, and discharge planning. To facilitate optimal collaboration with physician colleagues, nurses must understand HF pathophysiology, treatment strategies, and performance measures so they can augment and optimize care. Although there were no reports that compared nurse caregiver type, discussed using an advance practice nurse in the short-stay setting as a primary care provider, or assessed emergency care nurse caregiver knowledge of patient education principles, a few points can be made: (a) a team approach may meet the needs of patients with chronic HF better than an approach in which the emergency care physician is the sole short stay unit provider; (b) nurses with advanced degrees, skills, and training are capable of being a primary care provider in the management of chronically ill patients with HF once the diagnosis of decompensated HF has been made and the patient is deemed stable enough to allow for short stay care; and (c) emergency care nurses may require new (ongoing) knowledge to meet performance measures in HF pathophysiology, assessment, management, and patient education.

To facilitate the application of guidelines and performance measures, clinical leadership should be sought. This can be in the form of a cardiologist, HF specialty cardiologist, or advance practice nurse with HF specialty training. Changing and aligning the behavior of clinicians and managers will not be an easy task for the clinical leader. The ACC uses the Guidelines Applied in Practice (GAP) project and the AHA uses the Get with the Guidelines (GWTG) project to apply HF guidelines in practice. In both of these projects, effective clinical leadership is the key to achieving behavioral changes. Clinical leaders are center stage in motivating peers to achieve benchmarks for each performance measure and in influencing administration to provide resources that will facilitate goals.[21] When a clinical leader has a professional association with a national organization that ensures the scientific integrity of the recommendations for care, provides incentives for delivering optimal care, and aids in developing a leadership role, pressure for quality improvement intensifies and the need to manage change that supports the application of guidelines will be paramount.[21]

Part of the role of the clinical leader will be to structure the environment so that health care providers automatically deliver care that matches guideline recommendations. This requires tools that simplify and provide focus of HF care expectations by embedding evidence-based care into the care itself. In a HF management program for a short stay unit, some examples are as follows: preprinted HF admission order set; preprinted HF discharge planning checklist; HF discharge sheet; HF medication therapies list that includes the right drugs in each class, dosage steps from initial to target dosing, side and adverse effects, contraindications, and associated electrolyte monitoring; patient education handouts/booklet or video; and performance improvement prospective data collection flowsheets for assessment and medication administration. As noted earlier, availability of tools is not enough; they must be used by all health care providers and supported by institutional management.[4,21] Examples of tools are available in the ACC/AHA Clinical Performance Measures document[3] and through the GAP and GWTG projects.

A multidisciplinary team can provide patient support at a cost. Other professional caregivers that may benefit a short-stay HF management program are a pharmacist, social worker, gerontologist, echocardiographer, case manager, and nutritionist. Personnel resources allow nurses and physicians more time to focus on immediate HF care needs while knowing that psychosocial, economic, cultural, and other needs are being met by skilled team members. It is unknown whether using skilled multidisciplinary team members to deliver HF management or deal with issues associated with HF management adherence in a short stay unit leads to improvement in quality HF care or clinical outcomes such as reduced rehospitalization, improved quality of life, or improved adherence to self-care behaviors.

FACILITIES REQUIREMENTS

To achieve benchmark scores for the performance measures outlined in Table 8–1, facility requirements or enhancements may be needed, based on current operations and resources. Rationale for facility requirements is provided in Table 8–1.

Equipment for appropriate assessment is necessary for optimal investigation of diagnosis or HF cause, especially for echocardiography, B-type natriuretic peptide (BNP) laboratory testing, electrocardiography, and radiology. It is not necessary that the HF management program have exclusive use of equipment. Equipment can be shared by multiple departments or care providers can be sent to the short-stay area to perform services, as needed. Specialized equipment availability may not be needed around the clock because the patient is treated for a 23-hour period; however, delays in testing could lead to misdiagnosis, mismanagement, misappropriation of patient disposition, and increased cost of care. Table 8–3 lists ancillary facility resources that can benefit health care providers in care planning and implementation.

Materials that augment patient education and forms/algorithms that promote health care provider delivery of medical treatments should be developed, readily available for use, and consistently used by team members when patients meet criteria. Patient education materials (paper, video, and telehealth materials) can be costly when purchased from a vendor, and they may not be up-to-date with guideline recommendations. Developing patient education materials in-house requires attention to reading level; use of pictures, color, and formatting to make specific messages stand out; study of content for simplicity, accuracy, and thoroughness (including information on prognosis); and messages about who to contact for a variety of needs. In-house development can also be expensive, especially if the number of orders placed per shipment is low and/or health care providers or service availability is frequently altered.

Prespecified forms can augment documentation of routinely performed activities and remind providers of care expectations related to performance measures. When knowledgeable personnel use prespecified forms and algorithms to advance care and ensure care consistency, patients benefit by receiving optimal care and the system benefits by meeting or exceeding care expectations known to improve quality of care, morbidity, and

TABLE 8–3 **Ancillary Facility Resources That May Be Considered**

Resources	Purpose
Impedance cardiography	Hemodynamic assessment and monitoring during aggressive management
Electrocardiogram with S_3 and S_4 phonocardiogram features	Assessment of S_3 (diastolic volume overload) and S_4 (systolic ventricular overload)
Written care algorithms developed for specific interventions or situations	Promotes nurse-mediated care that can increase efficiency and throughput
Small videocassette or digital video player	Patients learn more easily via demonstration. Some patient education videos use demonstration to teach education principles
Patient care cubicle/room signs	Aids health care professionals to recognize patient limitations and/or care activities so that any encounter with a patient can be maximized (i.e., record intake and output, 2,000-mg sodium diet, fluid restriction of 2 L, weight before discharge)
Computer with web capabilities and printer to review and print heart failure data from a patient's internal hemodynamic monitor or implantable cardioverter defibrillator	Patients can download data from an implantable pacemaker type device from their home, over normal telephone lines. Access to data provides objective evidence of current condition that can be used in determining diagnosis, treatment plan, and prognosis.

mortality. Patient education and health care provider forms may require the services of a dedicated person or team to develop and revise content and maintain supplies. In addition, special computer software may be needed to create materials.

Facilities requirements must include systems that promote routine influenza and pneumococcal vaccination, documentation of assessment and treatments (signs and symptoms; laboratory testing; weight; functional status; medication classes, dosage, and side effects), documentation of patient education delivered, and documentation of delivered care compared with performance measure quality benchmarks. A quality monitor coordinator can devote time to chart review, data collection and entry of data into an electronic database, communication of outcomes, and replanning of services to enhance outcomes, as needed. There is no evidence that using a dedicated nurse or other professional person to promote evidence-based practice in a short-stay setting leads to enhanced performance or promotes patient health beyond what can be accomplished by training all nurses and other personnel working in the unit. Strengthening all personnel's level of understanding of HF principles is a first step in ensuring consistent communication, care delivery, and documentation of care delivery so that redundancies in care and billing can be eliminated. When a team approach is used, sharing of data, accountabilities, health care provider patterns, and finances can be shared and reviewed more critically.

SUMMARY

There are many gaps in best practice in regard to implementing a short-stay HF management program. Performance expectations need to be adapted from in-patient and ambulatory measures and modified to match the setting. It will be important to conduct research on performance measures in a short-stay environment so that standards of care are tailored to this setting. Staffing requirements include a clinical HF leader who can champion the program not just during development but over time. Other staffing requirements consistent with best practice suggest that knowledgeable nurses can augment physician care and that both physicians and nurses require education in HF, at least initially. Facilities resources can not only improve throughput for patients but also optimize care services that improve health care provider assessment, diagnosis, and management capabilities. Availability of well-developed patient education materials can enhance patient knowledge and improve self-care after discharge. A well-developed HF management program will have given considerable attention to performance measures, staffing, and facilities resources before program implementation.

REFERENCES

1. Joint Commission on Accreditation of Healthcare Organizations. Overview of the heart failure core measure set (3/22/2002). Available at http://jcaho.org/pms/core+measures/hf_overview.htm (accessed September 23, 2005).
2. Fonorow G, Abraham W, Albert N, et al. Should beta blocker use at the time of hospital discharge be included as a heart failure performance measure? A report from OPTIMIZE-HF. *J Cardiac Fail* 2005;11[Suppl]:S182.
3. American College of Cardiology/American Heart Association Task Force on Performance Measures. ACC/AHA clinical performance measures for adults with chronic heart failure. *J Am Coll Cardiol* 2005;46:1144–1178.
4. Ennis S, Moore S, Zichitella G, et al. Impact of a dedicated in-patient heart failure program on JCAHO core measures of heart failure care. *J Cardiac Fail* 2005;11[Suppl]:S183.
5. Joint Commission on Accreditation of Healthcare Organizations. Disease specific care. Request for public comment on disease-specific care standardized heart failure measure set. Available at http://jcaho.org/dscc/dsc/performance+measures/heart+failure+measure+set.htm (accessed September 23, 2005).
6. Peacock WF 4th, Remer EE, Aponte J, et al. Effective observation unit treatment of decompensated heart failure. *Congest Heart Fail* 2002;8:68–73.
7. Storrow AB, Collins SP, Lyons MS, et al. Emergency department observation of heart failure: preliminary analysis of safety and cost. *Congest Heart Fail* 2002;11:68–2.
8. Ansari M, Alexander M, Tutar A, et al. Cardiology participation improves outcomes in patients with new-onset heart failure in the outpatient setting. *J Am Coll Cardiol* 2003;41:62–68.

9. Jong P, Gong Y, Liu PP, et al. Care and outcomes of patients newly hospitalized for heart failure in the community treated by cardiologists compared with other specialists. *Circulation* 2003;108:184–191.

10. Reis SE, Holubkov R, Edmundowicz D, et al. Treatment of patients admitted to the hospital with congestive heart failure: specialty-related disparities in practice patterns and outcomes. *J Am Coll Cardiol* 1997;30:733–738.

11. Edep ME, Shah NB, Tateo IM, Massie BM. Differences between primary care physicians and cardiologists in management of congestive heart failure: relation to practice guidelines. *J Am Coll Cardiol* 1997;30:518–526.

12. Bello D, Shah NB, Edep ME, et al. Self-reported differences between cardiologists and heart failure specialists in the management of chronic heart failure. *Am Heart J* 1999;138:100–107.

13. Baker DW, Hayes RP, Massie BM, Craig CA. Variations in family physicians' and cardiologists' care for patients with heart failure. *Am Heart J* 1999;138:826–834.

14. Indridason OS, Coffman CJ, Oddone EZ. Is care associated with improved survival of patients with congestive heart failure? *Am Heart J* 2003;145:300–309.

15. Khunti K, Hearnshaw H, Baker R, Grimshaw G. Heart failure in primary care: qualitative study of current management and perceived obstacles to evidence-based diagnosis and management by general practitioners. *Eur J Heart Fail* 2002;4:771–777.

16. Whellan DJ, Gaulden L, Gattis WA, et al. The benefit of implementing a heart failure disease management program. *Arch Intern Med* 2001;161:2223–2228.

17. Smith LE, Fabbri SA, Pai R, et al. Symptomatic improvement and reduced hospitalization for patients attending a cardiomyopathy clinic. *Clin Cardiol* 1997;20:949–954.

18. Capomolla S, Febo O, Ceresa M, et al. Cost/utility ratio in chronic heart failure: comparison between heart failure management program delivered by day-hospital and usual care. *J Am Coll Cardiol* 2002;40:1259–1266.

19. Eliaszadeh P, Yarmohammadi H, Nawaz H, et al. Congestive heart failure case management: a fiscal analysis. *Dis Manage* 2001;4:25–32.

20. Albert NM, Collier S, Sumodi V, et al. Nurses' knowledge of heart failure education principles. *Heart Lung* 2002;31:102–112.

21. Eagle KA, Garson AJ, Beller GA, Sennett C. Closing the gap between science and practice: the need for professional leadership. *Health Affairs* 2003;22:196–201.

22. Hunt SA, Abraham WT, Chin MH, et al. ACC/AHA 2005 guideline update for the diagnosis and management of chronic heart failure in the adult: a report of the American College of Cardiology/American Heart Association Task Force on Practical Guidelines. Available at http://www.acc.org/clinical/guidelines/failure/index.pdf (accessed August 17, 2005).

23. Koelling TM, Johnson ML, Cody RJ, Aaronson KD. Discharge education improves clinical outcomes in patients with chronic heart failure. *Circulation* 2005;111:179–185.

24. American Heart Association. *Heart disease and stroke statistics—2005 update.* Dallas, TX: American Heart Association, 2004.

25. Shivkumar K, Jafri SM, Gheorghiade M. Antithrombotic therapy in atrial fibrillation: a review of randomized trials with special reference to the Stroke Prevention in Atrial Fibrillation II (SPAF II) Trial. *Prog Cardiovasc Dis* 1996;38:337–342.

26. Rame JE, Sheffield MA, Dires DL, et al. Outcomes after emergency department discharge with a primary diagnosis of heart failure. *Am Heart J* 2001;142:714–719.

27. Gattis WA, O'Connor CM, Gallup DS, et al. Predischarge initiation of carvedilol in patients hospitalized for decompensated heart failure: results of the Initiation Management Predischarge: Process for Assessment of Carvedilol Therapy in Heart Failure (IMPACT-HF) trial. *J Am Coll Cardiol* 2004;43:1534–1541.

28. Mueller C, Scholer A, Laule-Kilian K. Use of B-type natriuretic peptide in the evaluation and management of acute dyspnea. *N Engl J Med* 2004;350:647–654.

9

EMERGENCY DEPARTMENT AND OBSERVATION UNIT DISCHARGE CRITERIA

Deborah B. Diercks

Heart failure (HF) causes substantial morbidity and mortality in the United States and is the most common principal discharge diagnosis in adults aged 65 years and older.[1-3] Altogether, the costs for HF hospitalizations are approximately $14.7 billion per year.[4] A substantial number of these patients present to the emergency department for the initial treatment of their acute decompensation. It has been suggested that 80% of all patients who present with acute decompensated heart failure (ADHF) are admitted to the hospital.[5] Identifying patients who are suitable for discharge home or for admission to an observation unit (OU) may substantially reduce overall hospital costs. However, for emergency physicians, accurate disposition is a challenge and perhaps more daunting than the management of these patients.

Disposition decisions are often time-dependent and lack adequate time to assess response to treatment. This may result in inappropriate admissions and premature emergency department (ED) discharges, with resultant increased cost and morbidity, respectively.[6,7] Although the American College of Cardiology (ACC)/American Heart Association (AHA) guidelines on the management of HF suggest that patients with mild to moderate symptoms generally do not require admission, risk assessment based on symptoms is often difficult.[5] To increase the number of patients discharged to home, effective treatment must be initiated in the ED as part of their ED management or an OU protocol. This early intervention and avoidance of hospital admission can result in significant cost savings, because 75% of costs arising from hospitalization for HF are incurred within the first 48 hours.[4]

Success of any protocol is dependent on accurate identification of patients suitable for an early discharge plan. Patients with a high probability of adverse outcome, such as those with evidence of acute cardiac ischemia, should be admitted to the hospital as in-patients. Blood pressure and heart rate are two of the most significant independent predictors of acute mortality in patients with ADHF;[8] thus, patients with unstable vital signs, including a heart rate greater than 130 beats per minute, systolic blood pressure (SBP) less than 85 mm Hg or greater than 175 mm Hg after initial ED treatment, and O_2 saturation less than 90%, are inappropriate for an early discharge strategy.[9] In addition, patients with airway instability, inadequate systemic perfusion, or cardiac arrhythmias requiring continuous intravenous (IV) intervention, as well as those requiring invasive hemodynamic monitoring or receiving medications that require frequent uptitration, such as nitroglycerin, are also not suitable for an HF OU admission.[9]

As essential as the identification of appropriate patients for this rapid treatment protocol is, use of discharge criteria to result in a low rate of subsequent hospital readmission soon after discharge is also important. Unfortunately, there is a paucity of data addressing this issue in the ED, in-patient, and OU settings. Current methods of risk stratification have focused on identifying patients at risk for short- and long-term adverse events. Risk stratification is an ongoing process. It is dependent on clinical appearance, laboratory parameters, and response to acute therapies. Discharge to home should be considered from the perspective of an estimate of the acuity of the initial presentation of the patient, improvement in response to treatment, and risk of recidivism after discharge. It is suggested that certain clinical features should then alter the physician's initial acuity estimate and improvement in these parameters can identify patients suitable for discharge to home.

Consensus guidelines for discharge from the ED and OU have been developed.[10] These guidelines are based on the presence of factors associated with increased risk for adverse events. Although the absence of these parameters does not ensure that a patient is ready for discharge, they are useful in identifying patients with persistent decompensated HF who would benefit from additional treatment. These discharge criteria can be divided into three categories: patient-centered measures, hemodynamic and clinical parameters, and laboratory results (Table 9-1).

It has been well established that patient-centered outcome measures, such as a change in dyspnea, can be used to assess therapeutic success and improvement in symptoms. Although subjective, the measurement of dyspnea on a seven-point or three-point scale is a validated outcome measure.[11] In addition, the assessment of dyspnea has been shown to correlate with hemodynamic status in clinical trials. However, no study has evaluated this as an endpoint in an ED or OU, although it continues to be assessed in informal manners.[11] Another patient-centered measure that should be present at the time of discharge is the lack of ongoing chest pain. It has been reported that acute coronary syndrome (ACS) is a trigger for up to 25% of HF decompensation. Therefore, patients should be pain free or have undergone an evaluation for ACS prior to discharge.[12] Finally, the patient should be able to ambulate without an increase in dyspnea from baseline. Although no trial has assessed this measure in an OU setting, it effectively is an inexpensive 6-minute exercise test. The distance that

TABLE 9–1 Discharge Criteria

Patient Measures
No chest pain that would raise concern for acute coronary syndrome (ACS)[12]
Improvement in dyspnea[11]
Ability to ambulate without dyspnea above baseline[13]
Free of symptoms of congestion[14]
Hemodynamic/Clinical Parameters
SBP <160 mm Hg, >90 mm Hg[15]
No S_3 on auscultation[16]
Improvement in thoracic electrical bioimpedance measurements[19]
Oxygen saturation >90%[10]
Urine output >1 L[10]
Decrease in weight/return to dry weight
Laboratory Results
BNP levels[17-19]
Stable creatinine[17]
Stable or declining troponin level[20]
Return to normal or baseline of electrolytes and blood urea nitrogen (BUN)[22]

BNP, B-type natriuretic peptide; SBP, systolic blood pressure.

a patient can ambulate in a 6-minute period without excessive dyspnea and fatigue has been shown to correlate with long-term mortality. Unfortunately, many comorbid illnesses, such as obesity and lung disease, affect this outcome measure; hence, it is important to assess a change from baseline.[13] In addition, freedom from symptoms of congestion such as orthopnea has also been associated with improved long-term outcomes.[14]

Hemodynamic and clinical parameters can also be used as part of the data to assess suitability for discharge. These comprise measures of perfusion, volume status, and oxygenation based physical examination findings and automated measures. SBP is a useful predictor of adverse events at the time of presentation and discharge.[15] In the initial presentation of patients with decompensated HF, a hypertensive response is adaptive; however, persistent elevation of SBP can correlate with increased risk of worsening renal function. This deterioration of renal function clearly correlates with morbidity and mortality; therefore, adjustment of medications to prevent hypertension is essential prior to discharge. Although the ideal blood pressure at the time of hospital discharge is not clearly elucidated, patients should at least have an SBP less than 160 mm Hg.[15] In addition, as medications are titrated patients must be able to ambulate without symptoms of dizziness; therefore, patients should have an SBP greater than 90 mm Hg.[10]

Clinical findings can also be used to assess adequacy of acute interventions. These include a combination of changes in physical examination findings and easily obtained values, such as pulse oximetry, weight, and urine output. Of all the clinical examination findings, the presence of an S_3 is most suggestive of acute decompensation.[16] Serial examinations that can document the resolution of an S_3 can be used as a discharge criteria.[16] This physical examination finding, like an improvement in jugular venous distention, is dependent on physical attributes of the patient and careful physical examination assessment by the physician. Another criterion noted as part of the evaluation is oxygen saturation. Patients should have an oxygen saturation greater than 90%.[10] No data exist to support this value; however, it is reasonable to discharge only patients who are able to maintain their oxygen saturation. Transient nighttime drops in oxygen saturation are common because HF is associated with an increased prevalence of obstructive sleep apnea. Therefore, pulse oximetry as a discharge criterion should be assessed when the patient is awake.

Urine output assessment is another parameter that can be used as a surrogate to assess treatment efficacy. Although there are no studies that compare the amount of urine output with outcomes, intuitively this makes sense. Clinically, 1 liter (L) appears to be a significant amount. Closely linked to urine output is a decline in patient weight.[10] Dry weight is often one of the only baseline parameters that we know in the ED. Theoretically, a decline in the patient's weight can represent a resolution of the acute progression of the disease process; however, overshooting this parameter can lead to hypotension, hypoperfusion, and worsening renal function. Although not supported by clinical trials, it is reasonable to suggest that a patient's weight should be declining at the time of discharge; however, additional assessment may be warranted in patients who are below their dry weight at the time of discharge.

Improvement in laboratory results may be used to assess patients at the time of discharge. Studies have shown that a decline in B-type natriuretic peptide (BNP) levels is associated with improved morbidity and decreased hospital readmission rate.[17–19] However, no study has looked at the change in BNP levels in the less than 23-hour timeframe. It makes intuitive sense that a patient's BNP should be declining at the time of discharge assessment, although the exact amount of decline is unknown. Elevated troponin levels have been shown to be predictive of long-term prognosis in HF patients.[20] Patients with severe HF may have chronically elevated levels. However, a rise in troponin levels during an OU stay should provoke concern and may reflect inadequacy of treatment or the presence of ACS. In addition, patients with an elevated initial troponin level have been shown to be more likely to stay in the hospital greater than 24 hours and have a high rate of 30-day hospital readmission.[21] Therefore, patients with an elevated initial troponin level are probably not suitable for an early discharge strategy.

Traditional chemistry laboratory tests that are routinely assessed daily in patients with decompensated HF can also be used in the assessment of a patient at the time of discharge. A sodium level of less than 136 mEq/L and a serum blood urea nitrogen (BUN) greater than 43 mg/dL have been shown to correlate with 1-year and acute mortality, respectively.[8,22] Therefore, improvement in the BUN and serum creatinine in patients with abnormal values is a potential marker of treatment success and may be useful in determining disposition.[23] At this point, there are no trials that have used these values in this capacity. Recently, a significant amount of attention has been placed on the significance of worsening serum creatinine in the setting of treatment for decompensated HF. A recent study has shown that an increase in creatinine level of greater than 0.3 mg/dL from hospital admission correlates with greater rates of in-hospital death, increased complications, and longer length of stay. The presence of worsening renal insufficiency as defined by a creatinine change greater than 0.3 mg/dL from prior values is concerning, and therefore patients warrant further treatment until the creatinine improves or stabilizes.[24]

Independent of the clinical presentation, the success of early discharge is dependent on adequate outpatient follow-up and appropriate medication adjustment at the time of discharge. The initial improvements gained in the ED or OU can be quickly negated if the patient is discharged without a suitable outpatient management plan. Key components include close follow-up to ensure adequate medication adjustment, dietary education, and a management plan (Table 9-2). An important component of outpatient HF disease management includes[25,26] a cohesive management plan, which has been shown to result in a 25% to 75% reduction in hospitalization.[27,28]

Optimizing the medical regimen is another complex portion of the disposition process, because it requires coordination among many providers, including the treating ED physician, OU treating physician, consultants, and the outpatient provider. Although beyond the scope of this chapter, medication considerations should include the titration of loop diuretic, spironolactone, angiotensin-converting enzyme inhibitor, beta-blockers, and possibly nitrates.[25,26]

It should also be noted that every patient will not fit every criterion and that every recommendation must be interpreted with the patient's

TABLE 9–2 Outpatient Key Components

Nursing case management

Physician follow-up (primary care coordinated with cardiology)

Optimization of medication regimen

Patient education

Social support (home health assessment)

baseline status as well as their follow-up care in mind. The best recommendations contain a combination of these mentioned parameters adjusted for the individual patient. Using a combination of patient-centered outcomes and more objective measures provides ample evidence that can help drive the disposition decision. Appropriate discharge from the emergency room or OU must be accompanied with adequate follow-up. Also extremely important is patient education on dietary recommendations, medication schedules, and tracking body weight to help prevent the need for further emergency room visits or hospital admissions.

REFERENCES

1. Massie BM, Shah NB. Evolving trends in the epidemiologic factors of heart failure: rationale for preventive strategies and comprehensive disease management. *Am Heart J* 1997;133:703–712.
2. Rich MW. Epidemiology, pathophysiology, and etiology of congestive heart failure in older adults. *J Am Geriatr Soc* 1997;45:968–974.
3. Haldeman GA, Croft JB, Giles WH, et al. Hospitalization of patients with heart failure: National Hospital Discharge Survey, 1985 to 1995. *Am Heart J* 1999;137:352–360.
4. American Heart Association, American Stroke Association. *Heart disease and stroke statistics 2004 update.* Available at http://www.americanheart.org/downloadable/heart/1072969766940HSStats2004Update.pdf (accessed May 15, 2005).
5. Hunt SA, Baker DW, Chin MH, et al. ACC/AHA guidelines for the evaluation and management of chronic heart failure in the adult. *J Am Coll Cardiol* 2001;38:2101–2113.
6. Kosecoff J, Kahn KL, Rogers WH, et al. Prospective payment system and the impairment at discharge: the "quicker and sicker" story revisited. *JAMA* 1990;264:1980–1983.
7. Peacock WF IV, Remer ER, Aponte J, et al. Effective observation unit treatment of decompensated heart failure. *Congest Heart Fail* 2002;8:68–73.
8. Fonarow GC, Adams KF Jr, Abraham WT, et al. Risk stratification for in-hospital mortality in acutely decompensated heart failure: classification and regression tree analysis. *JAMA* 2005;293:572–580.
9. Peacock WF, Emerman CL, on behalf of the PROACTION Study Group. Safety and efficacy of nesiritide in the treatment of decompensated heart failure in observation patients [abstract 1027-89]. *J Am Coll Cardiol* 2003;41[Suppl A]:336A.
10. Cleveland Clinic. Management of acute decompensated heart failure in the emergency department. Available at http://www.clevelandclinicmeded.com/hfed/disch_guide.htm (accessed June 14, 2004).
11. Teerlink JR. Dyspnea as an end point in clinical trials of therapies for acute decompensated heart failure [review]. *Am Heart J* 2003;145[Suppl 2]:S26–S33.
12. Khand AU, Gemmell I, Rankin AC, Cleland JG. Clinical events leading to the progression of heart failure: insights from a national database of hospital discharges. *Eur Heart J* 2001;22:153–164.
13. Rostagno C, Olivo G, Comeglio M, et al. Prognostic value of 6-minute walk corridor test in patients with mild to moderate heart failure: comparison with other methods of functional evaluation. *Eur J Heart Fail* 2003;5:247–252.
14. Luca C, Johnson W, Hamilton MA, et al. Freedom from congestion predicts good survival despite previous class IV symptoms of heart failure. *Am Heart J* 2000;140:840–847.
15. Forman DE, Butler J, Wang Y, et al. Incidence, predictors at admission, and impact of worsening renal function among patients hospitalized with heart failure. *J Am Coll Cardiol* 2004;43:61–67.

16. Marantz PR, Kaplan MC, Alderman MH. Clinical diagnosis of congestive heart failure in patients with acute dyspnea. *Chest* 1990;97:776–781.

17. Cheng V, Kazanagra R, Garcia A, et al. A rapid bedside test for B-type peptide predicts treatment outcomes in patients admitted for decompensated heart failure: a pilot study. *J Am Coll Cardiol* 2001;37:386–391.

18. Knebel F, Schimke I, Pliet K, et al. NT-ProBNP in acute heart failure: correlation with invasively measured hemodynamic parameters during recompensation. *J Card Fail* 2005;11[5 Suppl]:S38–41.

19. Kazanegra R, Cheng V, Garcia A, et al. A rapid test for B-type natriuretic peptide correlates with falling wedge pressures in patients treated for decompensated heart failure: a pilot study. *J Card Fail* 2001;7:21–29.

20. Potluri S, Ventura HO, Mulumudi M, Mehra MR. Cardiac troponin levels in heart failure. *Cardiol Rev* 2004;12:21–25.

21. Diercks DB, Peacock WF, Kirk JD, Weber JE. Emergency department heart failure patients: identification of an observational unit appropriate cohort. *J Card Fail* 2004(abst).

22. Felker GM, Leimberger JD, Califf RM, et al. Risk stratification after hospitalization for decompensated heart failure. *J Card Fail* 2004;10:460–466.

23. Lee DS, Austin PC, Rouleau JL, et al. Predicting mortality among patients hospitalized for heart failure: derivation and validation of a clinical model. *JAMA* 2003;290:2581–2587.

24. Forman DE, Butler J, Wang Y, et al. Incidence, predictors at admission, and impact of worsening renal function among patients hospitalized with heart failure. *J Am Coll Cardiol* 2004;43:61–67.

25. Nohria A, Lewis E, Stevenson LW. Medical management of heart failure. *JAMA* 2002;287:628–640.

26. Peacock WF 4th. Rapid optimization: strategies for optimal care of decompensated congestive heart failure patients in the emergency department. *Rev Cardiovasc Med* 2002;3[Suppl 4]:S41–S48.

27. Rich MW, Beckham V, Wittenberg C, et al. A multidisciplinary intervention to prevent the readmission of elderly patients with congestive heart failure. *N Engl J Med* 1995;333:1190–1195.

28. Hanumanthu S, Butler J, Chomsky D, et al. Effect of a heart failure program on hospitalization frequency and exercise tolerance. *Circulation* 1997;96:2842–2848.

10

THE ESSENTIALS OF PATIENT EDUCATION IN THE EMERGENCY DEPARTMENT

Robin J. Trupp and Elsie M. Selby

INTRODUCTION

Heart failure is a complex chronic condition associated with great morbidity, mortality, and economic burden in the United States. The vast majority of health care expenses related to heart failure occur as a result of hospitalizations for decompensation.[1] Identification of the reason for the decompensation, such as further deterioration in left ventricular function or a remedial cause, determines the treatment plan. Importantly, in most instances, these hospitalizations could be avoided with adherence to treatment regimens and/or careful monitoring and attention to changes in signs and symptoms of heart failure.[2-4] Although educational needs for the patient with heart failure are vast and include such topics as the pathophysiology and etiology of heart failure and necessary lifestyle modifications, in an observation unit education must be directed and succinct, given the short-term nature of the interaction. However, during times of stress, as would be expected in patients presenting to an emergency department, retention of any information given is limited.[5] If the patient is ultimately hospitalized, the urgency for providing information is somewhat lessened, because the inpatient environment offers additional opportunity for, and reinforcement of, education. Because the majority of causes of worsening heart failure are directly attributable to nonadherence to the medication and/or dietary regimens, this chapter concentrates on these topics as essential elements of patient education.

Adherence to prescribed medical regimens, including both pharmacologic and nonpharmacologic interventions, significantly impacts both the short- and long-term management of heart failure. Such treatment strategies have been well proven to slow disease progression, reduce hospital admissions, and improve overall symptom control.[6] However, despite the importance of these interventions, numerous barriers to adherence exist. Barriers may include lack of understanding of perceived benefit, lifestyle modifications, absence of social support, powerlessness, financial concerns, and time constraints. These barriers complicate patients' ability and willingness to adhere to the prescribed medical regimen. In addition, in the haste to shorten length of stay and reduce health care expenditures, clinicians may simply treat the symptoms and fail to identify nonmedical causes for the decompensation. By taking the time to do a thorough assessment to identify barriers and then target problem areas, clinicians can better use the time spent with each patient, leading to a more individualized treatment plan and enhanced adherence.[7]

CAUSES FOR DECOMPENSATION

Poor compliance with the medication regimen and volume overload, directly related to sodium indiscretion (willful or inadvertent) and/or excess fluid intake, are the major causes for decompensated, or worsening, heart failure.[3,8] In many of these instances, improved communication between the patient and health care team could have provided an opportunity to intervene and avoid hospitalization. Using an organized multidisciplinary team affords greater opportunities for achieving treatment goals and outcomes. The success of multidisciplinary teams is well documented in the medical and nursing literature, and much of their success is directly related to enhanced communication, improved adherence, and increased attention to early warning signs of worsening heart failure.

MEDICATION AND DIETARY ADHERENCE

Diet and medication adherence have profound implications for the management of heart failure. Lack of adherence as a significant cause of decompensation and hospitalization has been well documented.[3] Poor adherence also has significant economic repercussions. For example, if insufficient medication is taken for the treatment to be fully effective, as occurs when patients "ration" diuretics to extend the life of a prescription, subsequent health care costs are likely to be incurred as a result of hospital-based treatment. Not unexpectedly, better outcomes are seen with improved adherence to treatment plans.[6]

The role of education on medication and dietary adherence cannot be overemphasized and requires continual reinforcement. Clinicians working with heart failure patients are challenged to approach each patient as unique and to individualize strategies to increase adherence to diet and medication. One size does not fit all here.

Dietary Instructions

In general, sodium intake should be limited to about 2,000 mg per day for all patients with heart failure, regardless of type of dysfunction or the use of diuretics. Because the average American diet consists of approximately 6,000 mg per day, this degree of sodium restriction is challenging for even the most dedicated patient. Counseling should include repeated in-depth instruction on the components of a 2-g sodium diet and should involve family members as well. Although patients not suffering from advanced disease may be able to tolerate more sodium, limiting intake to 2,000 mg sodium daily is advised because consumption will likely exceed the recommendations anyway. Salt substitutes and spices may be used to improve the palatability of food. However, some salt substitutes replace sodium chloride with potassium chloride and should be used with caution, given the potential risk of hyperkalemia.

In advanced heart failure, further dietary sodium restriction may be necessary to attenuate expansion of extracellular fluid volume and the development of edema. Although sodium restriction may assuage the development of edema, it cannot totally prevent it, because the kidneys are capable of reducing urinary sodium excretion to less than 10 mmol per day. Hyponatremia should not discourage compliance with a restricted sodium diet, because the hyponatremia is usually dilutional in nature and associated with total body sodium and water excess. Liberalized sodium intake or replacement, therefore, should be considered only in overt cases of severe excessive diuresis and dehydration.

Within the emergency department, simple questions about recent dietary intake may yield the cause of decompensation. Accompanying family members are also good sources of information regarding food or fluid intake. Patients should understand the relationship between fluid and sodium for managing volume and in controlling symptoms. Instructing patients to simply take an extra diuretic to relieve symptoms should not be encouraged, because diuretics contribute to increased neurohormonal stimulation and worsening renal function.[7] Patients should understand that dietary indiscretion produces fluid retention and worsening symptoms. Thus, efforts should focus on helping patients make the association between behavior and symptoms. The challenge lies in doing this without preaching or condemning. Learning will not occur within that scenario. If a connection between a particular behavior and its negative consequences can be made, lifestyle changes are more likely. Behavioral changes do not happen overnight, but those who view the recommended changes as personal choices, rather than as edicts imposed by others, are more likely to make permanent lifestyle modifications.[8]

Recognizing obvious sources of sodium, such as the salt shaker or potato chips, is evident for most patients but in a typical diet constitutes less than 25% of total intake. Hidden sources of sodium play a major role in dietary intake yet are often unrecognized. Good heart failure clinicians are also good detectives. Common high-sodium-content items include, but are not limited to, canned soups and vegetables, pickles, cheese, softened water, tomato juice, antacids, and processed foods. Having the patient complete a food diary over the course of several days will give the clinician important insights into dietary habits and average fluid consumption and will likely reveal unexpected high-sodium sources. Starting this diary after treatment in the emergency department affords the clinician next evaluating the patient much-needed information and the ability to offer alternative lower sodium choices. Resources available for patients include pamphlets or booklets on the sodium content of foods, for use both at home and when dining out. These materials should be readily located and available within the emergency department. Another more commonly used resource is the Internet, where numerous web sites related to low-sodium food choices and recipes can be located.

Medications

Pharmacologic interventions are vital to managing symptoms and halting disease progression in heart failure. Yet, medications for heart failure are both complex and costly. Polypharmacy, or the need for multiple medications, is a normal consequence of an evidence-based approach to managing heart failure, because beta-blockers, angiotensin-converting enzyme (ACE) inhibitors and/or angiotensin receptor blockers, aldosterone inhibitors, electrolyte supplements, and diuretics must all be taken at different times throughout the day. No wonder patients become confused and fail to comply. Potential barriers to adherence should be identified and addressed. Besides financial barriers, other frequently missed obstacles include real or perceived side effects, forgetfulness, and understanding the importance of the medication.[5,6] To improve patient adherence, ongoing discussions must occur between clinicians and patients to reach understanding and agreement on the necessity for medications and the appropriate regimen.[6] Rather than mandated or imposed views, this discussion may require some compromise from both parties, as patients agree to take more medications than they initially wanted or as the clinician acknowledges the patient may be taking less than is ideal. What is most important is that the actual medications being taken are known.

Patients should be instructed to bring their medications whenever seeking or receiving health care. Doing so provides an accurate record of current medications and prevents duplicate prescriptions. A variety of aids to enhance adherence are available and may be helpful to some. These aids include pill boxes, medication trackers, or timers, to name few. For those with financial constraints, most major pharmaceutical companies offer assistance programs for individuals unable to afford medications. Documentation of medical necessity is required from the prescribing clinician, and patients may need to submit documentation of financial need as well. Although this process is unlikely to be initiated in the emergency department, it is important to recognize resource options and to make the necessary referrals.

WORSENING SIGNS AND SYMPTOMS

Despite advanced warning signs and symptoms of decompensation, many patients either fail to recognize them or fail to react. For example, Friedman reported that 90% of patients hospitalized due to decompensation experienced dyspnea 3 days prior to hospitalization.[9] Additionally, 35%

reported edema and 33% had cough 1 week prior to admission.[10] A survey by Carlson and Riegel[11] revealed that most patients had experienced multiple symptoms of worsening heart failure in the previous year, yet their knowledge of the importance of these signs and symptoms was poor. Even though patients who had lived with heart failure for years were more likely to use appropriate self-care strategies than newly diagnosed patients, they were uncomfortable in evaluating the effectiveness of their own actions.[11] Thus, when patients fail to recognize or acknowledge worsening signs and symptoms, clinicians lose the chance to intervene and potentially avert hospitalization. Therefore, educating patients and their families on both the signs and symptoms associated with worsening heart failure and what actions to take provides an excellent opportunity to reduce hospitalizations and ultimately reduce health care expenditures. Establishing self-efficacy, or belief in the ability to control heart failure, is essential for patients to participate in their own care and better manage their disease.

Patients experiencing decompensated heart failure exhibit a constellation of signs and symptoms, including increased dyspnea and/or fatigue, weight gain, orthopnea, and paroxysmal nocturnal dyspnea (PND). Essential aspects of education are presented in Table 10-1. Patients need simple advice on what changes in symptoms are important and clear endpoints that should prompt them to seek help. Whenever special equipment is involved, instruction on proper use and when to seek help are required. For example, daily weights require that the patient owns a scale, that the scale has numbers that can be read by the patient with a stable base large enough for them to stand on, and that the weights be obtained at approximately the same time each day. Education on when to call with weight changes is determined by the clinician and should be provided in written format and then reinforced frequently. In all cases, patients and families should be diligent in monitoring physical signs and symptoms. Establishing plans for notifying health care providers of any changes is the logical next step and should include the identification of emergency contact numbers for doing so.

Respiratory Symptoms

The majority of patients with decompensated heart failure have evidence of excess extracellular volume or congestive signs and symptoms. However, typical respiratory complaints, such as dyspnea, have poor sensitivity and are nonspecific to heart failure.[12] In addition, many patients with heart failure also have significant comorbidities that may further limit respiratory function, such as chronic pulmonary disease or obesity. When such comorbidities are present, the clinical importance of these alterations from everyday respiratory limitations becomes the measure for pending decompensation. For example, using three pillows to sleep may be a normal sleep pattern for some and should not be considered as evidence of orthopnea, but for others, a change from one pillow to two pillows may be indicative of worsening heart failure. Further questioning about sleep patterns can also

TABLE 10-1   **Essentials of Heart Failure Patient Education**

- **Daily weights every day of your life.**
  - √ Use the same scale at the same time of the day wearing comparable clothing.
  - √ Weigh first thing in the morning after going to the bathroom.
  - √ Notify your health care provider if you gain 3 or more pounds overnight or 5 pounds over 3 days OR if you lose weight and experience dizziness on standing up.

- **Maintain a low sodium diet to help avoid fluid retention.**
  - √ A dietary intake of 2,000 mg of sodium per day is recommended.
  - √ Ask for written materials to help you make healthier choices.
  - √ Salt is everywhere. Learn to read labels.

- **Be conscious of fluid intake.**
  - √ Do not drink 8 glasses of water per day if taking a diuretic (water pill). This defeats the purpose of that medication.
  - √ Drink small sips when thirsty or when taking medications.
  - √ Do not carry liquids with you.
  - √ Fluid comes in a variety of formats: soup, Jell-O, ice, watermelon.

- **Be as active as possible.**
  - √ Engage in physical activity at least 3–4 times per week.
  - √ Appropriate activities include walking or biking.

- **Avoid any form of heavy lifting or isometric exercises.**
  - (Isometric exercises are those in which a force is applied to a resistant object, such as pushing against a brick wall.)
  - √ Treatment of heart failure is directed at reducing the workload in your heart not straining it. Do not lift anything heavier than 10 pounds.

- **Notify your health care provider of changes in your symptoms or weight.**
  - √ This includes weight gain of 3 or more pounds overnight or 5 pounds over 3 days, increased fatigue or shortness of breath, dizziness, or fever, to name a few.
  - √ Your physician or nurse will give you additional, specific information to follow.
  - √ Keep their emergency number available in case of need.

provide additional insight. Patients may report sleeping on one pillow but fail to mention that one pillow is used in their recliner, because they cannot tolerate lying flat in bed without severe respiratory distress.

Patients with chronic heart failure live with dyspnea, and breathlessness becomes "normal" or a part of everyday life.[13] Adjustments to constant dyspnea usually center on reducing physical activities to reduce breathlessness. Seeking help occurs only when the usual strategies, such as rest or fresh air, fail to relieve symptoms and the patient becomes anxious or frightened. Initial treatment is aimed at rapidly alleviating the air hunger and hypoxia. It is important to remember that substantial pulmonary congestion can occur without rales or jugular venous pressure being evident.[14]

Changes in Weight

Just as diabetics monitor glucose levels to better manage their disease, so should heart failure patients monitor their weight. Daily weights comprise the gold standard for the outpatient care and management of heart failure and are indicated to permit the use of lower and safer doses of diuretics and for the titration of diuretics. As previously discussed, daily weights will not occur or be accurate if the patient does not own a scale, devalues the necessity of performing the task, or fails to do so consistently and appropriately.

Although the focus of weight monitoring is to detect weight gain, indicating fluid retention, patients should also pay attention to weight loss. Excessive weight loss can result in dehydration, electrolyte imbalances, or worsening renal function and produces symptoms of dizziness, fatigue, and shortness of breath. In advanced heart failure, when the patient's appetite and caloric intake decline, excess volume may take place in the absence of any apparent weight gain, as true body mass is lost through muscle and fat catabolism.

Fatigue

Patients with heart failure experience chronic fatigue and reduce their physical activity to mitigate exhaustion. However, worsening or increasing fatigue, in the absence of increased physical activity, can be an early indicator of decompensation. Any increased fatigue that lasts longer than 2 to 3 days should be a source of concern for the patient and should prompt closer attention to sodium and medication adherence. Should additional symptoms develop or the fatigue continue or worsen, health care providers should be notified immediately, to intervene and possibly avoid hospitalization. However, as with dyspnea, fatigue is a vague symptom that is difficult to quantify and can be included in the differential diagnosis for many other conditions and diseases.

Nocturia

One of the earliest symptoms of excess extracellular fluid is nocturia. To maintain homeostasis, the heart attempts to eliminate excess volume through the secretion of natriuretic peptides from the atrial and ventricular myocytes. These endogenous peptides act by dilating the renal afferent arteriole, preventing sodium reabsorption, and counteracting vasoconstriction effects. Atrial natriuretic peptide (ANP) is secreted primarily at night, when right atrial pressures are highest as a result of supine positioning. Consequently, urinary volume is increased, and the patient is awakened to void. Patients should pay attention to new onset or increasing nocturia that occurs in the absence of changes in the medication or dietary regimen.

REINFORCEMENT OF EDUCATION

Because high levels of relapse are likely to occur after short-term behavioral interventions, plans for reinforcement of the education must be established to improve long-term adherence and as relapse prevention.[15] Patients must be given instructions to schedule a follow-up visit with the primary care physician or other clinicians managing the heart failure within days of receiving treatment in the emergency room. This quick appointment serves two purposes. The first is to ensure that treatment has been adequate in resolving the patient's signs or symptoms and that no new issues have developed. Second, reinforcement of education can be provided, especially information specific to the cause of the decompensation. If the cause for the exacerbation was not identified, health care providers more familiar with the patient may be able to discern the cause at this appointment and provide the requisite education.

Because patients prefer information to be presented in different formats, a variety of educational materials must be accessible within the emergency department. Some examples of materials available include videotapes or CDs, pamphlets, or printed pages specifically printed and distributed by the institution. Having these materials at hand provides patients and families the opportunity to read and have questions answered, resulting in an expedited education process.

SUMMARY

For many, episodes of decompensated heart failure may be largely avoidable through self-monitoring of symptoms and enhanced adherence to treatment regimens. Unfortunately, during incidents of worsening heart failure, it can be difficult, if not impossible, to provide education to patients on better managing their disease. A better plan in the emergency department is to begin by treating the excess volume and alleviating the symptoms. Once stabilized and in the observation unit, there is an important opportunity and a teachable moment. Education and counseling that address specific concerns may provide the knowledge, support, and impetus to adherence to treatment plans and to recognize early signs of worsening heart failure and ultimately to reduce hospitalizations. Importantly, discharge instructions should include prompt follow-up with the established primary care physician. In advanced or complex cases, referral to a heart failure specialist is warranted.

REFERENCES

1. O'Connell JB, Bristow M. Economic impact of heart failure in the United States: time for a different approach. *J Heart Lung Transpl* 1994;13:107–112.

2. Evangelista LS, Dracup K. A closer look at compliance research in heart failure patients in the last decade. *Progr Cardiovasc Nurs* 2000;15(3):97–03.

3. Dunbar SB, Clark PC, Deaton C, et al. Family education and support interventions in heart failure. *Nurs Res* 2005;54(3):158–166.

4. Ni H, Nauman D, Donna Burgess D, et al. Factors influencing knowledge of and adherence to self-care among patients with heart failure. *Arch Intern Med* 1999;159:1613–1619.

5. Dominique JF, de Quervain DJF, Roozendaal B, et al. Acute cortisol administration impairs retrieval of long term declarative memory in humans. *Nat Neurosci* 2000;3:313–314.

6. Compliance or concordance: is there a difference? *Drugs Ther Perspect* 1999;13(1):11–12.

7. National Heart Lung and Blood Institute web site. NHLBI working group. Available at http://www.nhlbi.nih.gov/meetings.workshops.cardiorenal-hf-hd.htm (accessed August 16, 2005).

8. Ryan RH, Deci EL. Self-determination theory and the facilitation of intrinsic motivation, social development, and well-being. *Am Psychol* 2000;55:68–78.

9. Friedman M, Griffin JA. Relationship of physical symptoms and physical functioning to depression in patients with heart failure. *Heart Lung* 2001;30:98–104.

10. Vinson J, Chin MF, Goldman L. Factors contributing to the hospitalization of patients with congestive heart failure. *Am J Public Health* 1997;87:643–648.

11. Carlson B, Riegel B. Self-care abilities of patients with heart failure. *Heart Lung* 2001;30:351–359.

12. Maisel AD, Krishnaswany P, Nowak RM, et al. Rapid measurement of B-type natriuretic peptide in the emergency diagnosis of heart failure. *N Engl J Med* 2002;347:161–167.

13. Edmonds PE, Rogers A, Addington-Hall JM, et al. Patient descriptions of breathlessness in heart failure. *Int J Cardiol* 2005;98:61–66.

14. Young JB, Mills RM. *Clinical management of heart failure.* West Islip, NY: Professional Communications Inc, 2001.

15. Rutledge DN, Donaldson NE, Pravikoff DS. Patient education in disease and symptom management in congestive heart failure. *Online J Clin Innovations* 2001;15(2):1–52.

DISCHARGE PLANNING FOR HEART FAILURE IN THE SHORT STAY UNIT

Ginger A. Conway

SCOPE OF THE PROBLEM

Heart failure is the cause of nearly 1 million hospitalizations annually.[1-5] It is the most common discharge diagnosis among individuals aged 65 years and older, accounting for more than 640,000 discharges per year.[4-10] Readmissions have increased since the advent of the Medicare prospective payment system.[10] The 90-day readmission rates for individuals aged 70 years and older is between 40% and 60%.[2,11]

EMERGENCY DEPARTMENT TREATMENT OF PATIENTS WITH HEART FAILURE

Patients present to the emergency department (ED) expecting relief of their symptoms of heart failure. These patients are evaluated and treated and are then discharged to the outpatient setting or admitted to the hospital as necessary.[12] As many as 80% of those who present have previously been diagnosed with heart failure.[13] Many of these individuals can be successfully treated in the ED observation unit. This is a cost-saving approach but adds to the responsibility of the ED staff to provide comprehensive discharge planning.[13] Failure to meet this responsibility will result in repeated admissions to either the ED or the hospital. For those patients who go on to be admitted to the hospital, the assessment of discharge needs and the plan to meet these needs must begin in the ED.

WHAT IS DISCHARGE PLANNING?

Discharge planning is a process of evaluation of the patient's needs both during the admission and after discharge. It begins at the time of admission and must be re-evaluated and adjusted as needed several times during

117

the hospital stay.[11] The process involves an assessment of the precipitating factors resulting in the current admission, educational needs, and postdischarge care.[11,14] Discharge planning should involve the patient, all members of the health care team, the family, and any other caregivers with frequent collaboration.[11,14,15] The discharge planning process and the development of the plan should be documented in the patient's medical record.[14] The final plan should be communicated to the outpatient health care team, including the patient's primary care physician, because many readmissions occur due to the lack of communication between the pre- and postdischarge health care teams.[10,14,16]

A comprehensive, well-executed discharge planning process can prevent unnecessary delays in discharge and ensure that adequate support is available in the outpatient environment.[14,15] Effective discharge planning is necessary to decrease readmissions and is particularly beneficial for the elderly.[14,15] Inadequate discharge planning is linked to early unplanned readmissions.[17] Evidence of an effective discharge plan occurs when subsequent readmissions are not a result of the patient's or caregiver's misunderstanding of medications, diet, or exercise instructions.[16] The readmission also must not be related to lack of access to prescribed medications or treatments as a result of functional or financial limitations or psychosocial problems.[16]

WHO IS AT RISK FOR READMISSION?

Individuals who are at an increased risk for readmission need special attention during the discharge assessment and planning. Readmission rates are extremely high among all individuals with heart failure, with approximately 20% readmitted within 1 month of discharge and 50% within 6 months.[3,18-20] However, as many as 50% of readmissions might be prevented with comprehensive discharge planning and after-discharge follow-up.[11,21,22] Inadequate patient education and nonadherence to the medical plan may account for as many as 40% of the readmissions.[23]

Multiple factors have been associated with an increased risk for readmission. The elderly are at particularly increased risk, especially without adequate discharge planning.[21,24] They are often ill-prepared to make the necessary lifestyle changes that can improve outcomes.[24] All ages are at increased risk of readmission if they are inadequately prepared as a result of insufficient education and support prior to and after discharge.[21] Several physiologic risk factors have been identified (Table 11–1). When present, these risk factors indicate a greater chance that the patient will be readmitted to the hospital for care. Patients with these risk factors need increased attention to their discharge readiness.

Other contributing factors have to do with the patient's self-care measures and the ability to make the necessary lifestyle adjustments. Many patients fail to adhere to the medical plan due to lack of confidence

TABLE 11-1 **Physiologic Risk Factors for Readmission**[4,7,9,24,36,37]

Age 70 years or more	Edema at discharge
Ejection fraction < 35%	Weight loss of less than 3 kg
Ischemic etiology of heart failure	Serum creatinine 2.0 mg/dL or greater
History of renal failure	Systolic blood pressure >180 mm Hg
Diabetes mellitus	Diastolic blood pressure >100 mg Hg
Prior hospitalization in past 6 months	Lower serum sodium
Previous admission with length of stay greater than 7 days[32]	

that it is necessary or will help.[25] Many simply do not understand.[25] For instance, few patients have the knowledge of how to follow a low-sodium diet.[26] Noncompliance with medications and diet can lead to worsening symptoms and subsequent readmissions.[27,28] Butler et al.[20] reported that nearly one third of those discharged on an angiotensin-converting enzyme inhibitor (ACEI) stop taking them within 1 year. Delays in seeking medical care can also result in unnecessary readmissions.[28]

Nonadherence may result from conditions that are beyond the patient's control, such as cognitive impairments that may affect abilities to learn and comply. Forgetfulness or lack of interest and noncompliance with routine follow-up also contribute to readmissions.[27] The patient who is depressed is more likely to be readmitted.[25,27] The financial needs of the patient must be assessed.[11] The inability to pay for medications can negatively influence adherence. Many individuals have no prescription coverage, especially those older than 65 years who have Medicare as their sole source of insurance.[29] These individuals must pay out of pocket for their medications.[29] Hussey et al.[29] evaluated the charts of 138 patients with heart failure to determine chronic medications. The average number of medications taken by patients was 10.5. The number of medications increased as the severity of symptoms increased, and the mean monthly expenditure was $438.33.

The home environment can also have an effect. It is essential for the nurse to assess the level of involvement the family and outpatient support team are capable of and are willing to provide. The lack of adequate support at home can increase the likelihood of readmissions.[16,25]

IS THE PATIENT READY FOR DISCHARGE?

It is essential that the patient and the support team be adequately prepared for discharge. Kee and Borchers[16] reported that 40% to 59% of

TABLE 11–2 Physical Assessment[11,13]

Hemodynamic stability	Systolic BP >80 mm Hg
	Heart rate <100 beats/min
	Minimal orthostatic changes in BP
	Stable vital signs
	Oxygen saturation >90%
Cardiac rhythm	Stable
	No new significant arrhythmias
	No evidence ischemia
Renal function	Adequate urine output
	Electrolytes (within normal limits)
	Stable creatinine and BUN

BP, blood pressure; BUN, blood urea nitrogen.

admissions could be prevented with better assessment of readiness for discharge and adherence to guideline-based care. There are four areas that require assessment to determine discharge readiness. They are the physical condition of the patient, the medical plan, the patient's ability to comply, and the adequacy of support in the outpatient environment.

The physical examination needs to center around symptom improvement and hemodynamic stability, mobility, and renal function.[11,13] Patients should meet these physical parameters prior to discharge. Table 11–2 provides a list of parameters to be assessed. Also, patients who were ambulatory prior to admission should be able to ambulate without limiting orthostasis.

Medications need to be evaluated and adjusted prior to discharge. The preadmission medical plan should be reviewed for opportunities for improvement. One must try to determine if the admission was linked to a deficiency in the preadmission medication regimen. Lack of adherence to guideline-based care can increase readmissions. It is essential that the discharge plan include the prescription of medications that have strong evidence of improving outcomes and avoid medications that have a negative impact on outcomes. Table 11–3 lists some of the basic medication guidelines for chronic systolic heart failure. It is important not only that the patient be on the correct medications but also that the doses be optimized.[27] Butler et al.[20] reported that nearly half of heart failure patients are discharged from the hospital without a prescription of an ACEI. The medical treatment used to improve the patient's symptoms must be considered when deciding on the discharge medication plan.[11] The patient should also be made aware that the medical plan will need modifications after discharge.

TABLE 11-3 **Guidelines for Medications for Heart Failure Patients with Decreased Ejection Fraction**[38]

Class I		
ACEI	For all patients with current or prior symptoms	Level A
ARB	For those who are ACEI intolerant	Level A
Diuretics	For those with symptoms of fluid retention	Level C
Beta-blockers[a]	For stable patients	Level A
Aldosterone antagonist	For those with moderate to severe heart failure	Level B
Hydralazine and nitrate	For those on ACEIs and beta-blockers who have persistent symptoms	Level A
Class II		
Digoxin	For those with persistent symptoms despite being on Level A medications	Level B

ACEI, angiotensin-converting enzyme inhibitor; ARB, angiotensin receptor blocker. Class I: Conditions for which there is evidence and/or general agreement that a given therapy is beneficial, useful, and/or effective. Class II: Conditions for which there is conflicting evidence and/or divergence of opinion about the usefulness/efficacy of a therapy. Level A: Data are derived from multiple randomized clinical trials or meta-analyses. Level B: Data are derived from a single randomized trial, or nonrandomized studies. Level C: Consensus opinion of experts, case studies, or standard of care.
[a]Approved beta-blockers for heart failure (bisoprolol, carvedilol, and sustained-release metoprolol succinate).

IS THERE ADEQUATE SUPPORT AFTER DISCHARGE?

Time should be spent assessing the support needs of the patient after discharge. Lack of emotional support places the patient at greater risk for readmission.[25] The patient's caregivers should be involved in the assessment of needs and development of the plan.[14,25] Areas to be assessed include the general health status of the patient including the preadmission functional status and the needs for health services prior to admission.[11,14] The perceived needs from the caregiver's and the patient's points of view must be reviewed.[14] The patient, caregiver, and medical team should work together to establish goals for the patient's discharge, and a plan to meet the needs of the patient should be implemented. The postdischarge plan should include the timing and frequency of office visits and all necessary referrals to outpatient support services, such as home health care and a disease management program.[11,13]

EDUCATION NEEDS TO DECREASE RISKS OF READMISSION

The evaluation of the patient's preadmission health care behaviors including medication and dietary compliance should begin at the time of admission.[11,30]

Lack of knowledge about diet and medications is multifactorial and increases the risk of readmissions.[28,31] The resulting medication and dietary nonadherence leads to 48% to 50% of heart failure readmissions.[7,13,28,32] Medication adherence data indicate that 25% of patients skip medications.[31,32] Alarmingly, 38% of patients with heart failure report thinking they should drink large quantities of fluids and less than 50% indicate they avoid salty foods.[31]

Educational needs are unique to each individual, and the process of educating the patient should begin at the time of admission. The nurse must assess the patient's readiness to change. Potential triggers to change health care behavior include the patient's realization of the importance of the change as well as his or her energy level, physical condition, and current stressors.[33] The stress of the current admission for the symptoms of acute decompensated heart failure can limit the patient's ability to change. The desire may be there, but the ability may be lacking. It is essential that the nurse recognize the patient's readiness to change and adapt his or her expectations accordingly. The process of becoming ready to change will continue into the outpatient setting.[33]

One approach to successful education is a patient-centered approach that focuses on the patient's perceived needs.[30] Anthony and Hudson-Barr[30] reported that the patient's perceived educational needs do not necessarily match the needs identified by the health care team. Patients and providers agree on the importance of education about medications and side effects, but patients place greater preference on information regarding resumption of daily activities than do the health care providers.[30] The patient's perceived needs must be viewed as a priority and must be met for the patient to feel adequately prepared for discharge. Patients are also interested in learning about how to monitor their symptoms and progress as well as when and how to obtain assistance.[15] Delays in seeking care can contribute to readmissions.[28] They should also be taught about daily weights and how their symptoms relate to their self-care behaviors.[25] Being cognizant of the patient's self-identified needs and incorporating them in discharge planning may improve readiness for discharge.[30]

Patients prefer individualized patient-based instructions on new medications to the instructions they receive from their pharmacies. This is especially true among older patients. Suggestions for patient-centered educational tools included larger print, a schedule for taking the medications that is individualized to the specific patient's needs, and the purpose and possible side effects of the medication.[25,34] Education can ensure that the patient will get his or her prescriptions filled and will not stop taking their medications prematurely.[35] Use of prepared discharge materials on medications, lifestyle modifications, and symptom assessment can facilitate complete discharge instructions with less time.[30]

The education plan and progress need to be communicated with the patient's in-patient health care providers as well as the outpatient health care team.[14] The patient's caregivers and other outpatient support services need to be informed of the educational plan as well.[14] This should all be documented in the medical record. This documentation should include the patient's individual needs and progress as well as the outpatient caregiver's ability to follow through with the plan.[14] This plan should be continued in the outpatient setting. Patient education is a matter of standard of care, including specific elements on self-care behaviors, and has been identified as a quality indicator of comprehensive discharge education.[26]

Quality patient education not only is in the best interest of the patient but also has been mandated by the federal government. It is a required part of hospital discharge education and is now one of the core measures by which hospitals are evaluated.[34] There are many topics to review with the patient and the family. A preplanned educational program will prevent omissions in the patient's education. Table 11–4 provides a list of the most common topics to be reviewed.

TABLE 11–4   Topics of Discussion with Patient[27]

Disease process	Causes of heart failure and admissions
	Why symptoms occur
Self-care behaviors	Sodium and fluid restrictions
	Daily weight
	Symptom monitoring
	How and when to call for help
	Avoid smoking
	Avoid alcohol
Medications	Purpose
	Importance of adherence
	When to take
	Dose
	Side effects
Activity	How to assess tolerance
	Energy conservation techniques
Symptom assessment	Shortness of breath
	Orthopnea
	Paroxysmal nocturnal dyspnea
	Cough
	Nausea
	Abdominal bloating
	Early satiety
	Edema

DISCUSSION

Several studies have been published on the effects of a comprehensive discharge and follow-up plan for the hospitalized patient with heart failure. They have included interventions such as the use of specialty trained nurses, early intervention, and outpatient follow-up. Kleinpell and Gawlinski[19] reported that with the use of disease-specific discharge forms for heart failure and the use of advance practice nurses (APNs) in the in-patient setting they were able to significantly improve adherence to evidence-based guidelines and core measures including comprehensive discharge teaching.[19]

Klienpell[15] began discharge assessment and planning in the intensive care unit (ICU). Early assessment of discharge needs allowed for adequate time to plan for the home care needs, thus preventing delays at the time of discharge. They used the Discharge Planning Questionnaire (DPQ), which is a 51-item assessment of the patient's perceived needs after discharge. The patient was then asked to complete a Discharge Adequacy Rating Form after discharge to provide feedback to the investigators on the discharge planning. Their results indicated that beginning the discharge plan in the ICU was effective. The patients felt that the discharge planning was more comprehensive and that they were better prepared for their discharge. Specifically, they felt more confident about their knowledge of the medications and their ability to monitor their symptoms. However, on assessment 2 weeks after discharge, many elders did not remember the purpose and side effects of their medications,[15] thus reinforcing the need for repeated instructions in the outpatient setting. One additional advantage of postdischarge telephone follow-up may be that it provides an opportunity to assess for early warning signs of trouble.[15]

Schneider et al.[35] reported that the effectiveness of the verbal presentations, print material, problem-solving discussions during discharge planning, and medication instructions can decrease the likelihood of readmissions. Their efforts resulted in a statistically significant reduction in readmissions during a period up to 31 days postdischarge.[35]

Others have used alternative methods of discharge planning. Naylor et al.[14] reported the benefits of having a nurse available by telephone from the time of admission, through the hospitalization and continuing on for 2 weeks after the patient's discharge from the hospital. The nurse was available for questions related to the discharge plan from the family, patient, caregivers, and health care team. Other plans for telephone follow-up include making at least two phone calls to the patient. The first occurs within 24 to 48 hours of discharge and the second between 7 and 10 days. The purpose of these calls was to assess the patient's condition, answer any questions, and reinforce the discharge instructions.[14]

Koelling et al.[26] evaluated a 1-hour educational session provided by a nurse educator prior to discharge. The nurse provided written discharge information on medications, food and drug interactions, and side effects.

Other topics reviewed included dietary and fluid restrictions and common heart failure symptoms. Self-care behaviors such as daily weights, symptom monitoring, and when and how to call for help were also reviewed. The rationale for all the instructions was discussed.[26]

CONCLUSION

The ED short stay unit is the appropriate place to begin the evaluation of discharge needs and start the development of the discharge plan for all patients regardless of the planned disposition after the ED. Those who are going to be released from the ED back to their outpatient setting need comprehensive discharge planning. Assessments and interventions including education, individualized medication instruction and scheduling, dietary counseling, and outpatient care coordination that have been used in the in-patient setting may improve outcomes if implemented in the ED.

A variety of methods of postdischarge support have been evaluated. Specific interventions are often difficult to evaluate because of the multidisciplinary multiple-intervention approach in most programs. However, the evidence supports the need for a coordinated effort to prepare patients for discharge, beginning at the time of admission, with frequent evaluations. Appropriate individualized postdischarge care can have a positive impact on outcomes.

More research is needed to determine which interventions will yield the greatest benefit for the patient in this time of shorter and shorter stays for individuals seeking acute interventions for their heart failure symptoms.

REFERENCES

1. O'Connor CM, Stough WG, Gallup DS, et al. Demographics, clinical characteristics, and outcomes of patients hospitalized for decompensated heart failure: observations from the IMPACT-HF registry. *J Card Fail* 2005;11:200–205.
2. Capomolla S, Pinna G, LaRovere MT, et al. Heart failure case disease management program: a pilot study of home telemonitoring versus usual care. *Eur Heart J* 2004;6[Suppl F]:91–98.
3. Galbreath AD, Krasuski RA, Smith B. Long-term healthcare and cost outcomes of disease management in a large, randomized, community-based population with heart failure. *Circulation* 2004;110:3518–3526.
4. Adams KF, Fonarow GC, Emerman CL, et al. Characteristics and outcomes of patients hospitalized for heart failure in the United States: rationale, design and preliminary observations from the first 100,000 cases in the acute decompensated heart failure national registry (ADHERE). *Am Heart J* 2005;149: 209–216.
5. Dunagan WC, Littenberg B, Ewald GA, et al. Randomized trial of a nurse-administered, telephone-based disease management program for patients with heart failure. *J Card Fail* 2005;11:358–365.
6. Klienpell RM, Gawlinski A. Assessing outcomes in advance practice nursing. *AACN Clin Issues* 2005;19:43–67.
7. Rich MW, Beckham V, Wittenberg C, et al. A multidisciplinary intervention to prevent the readmission of elderly patients with congestive heart failure. *N Engl J Med* 1995;333: 1190–1195.

8. Stewart S, Pearson S, Horowitz JD. Effects of a home based intervention among patients with congestive heart failure discharged from an acute care hospital. *Arch Intern Med* 1998;158:1067–1072.

9. DiSalvo TG, Stevenson LW. Interdisciplinary team based management of heart failure. *Dis Manage Health Outcomes* 2003;11:87–94.

10. Phillips CO, Wright SM, Kern DE, et al. Comprehensive discharge planning with post-discharge support for older patients with congestive heart failure. *JAMA* 2004;291: 1358–1367.

11. Grady KL, Dracup K, Kennedy G, et al. Team management of patients with heart failure: a statement for healthcare professionals from the Cardiovascular Nursing Council of the American Heart Association. *Circulation* 2000;102:2443–2456.

12. Burkhardt J, Peacock WF, Ereman CL. Predictors of emergency department observation unit outcomes. *Acad Emerg Med* 2005;12:869–874.

13. Peacock WF. Emergency department observation unit management of heart failure. *Crit Pathways Cardiol* 2003;2:207–220.

14. Naylor M, Brooten D, Jones R, et al. Comprehensive discharge planning for the hospitalized elderly–a randomized clinical trial. *Ann Intern Med* 1994;120:999–1006.

15. Kleinpell RM. Randomized trial of an intensive care unit-based early discharge planning intervention for critically ill elderly patient. *Am J Crit Care* 2004;13:335–345.

16. Kee CC, Borchers L. Reducing readmission rates through discharge interventions. *Clin Nurse Spec* 1998;12:206–209.

17. Kossovsky MP, Sarasin FP, Perneger TV, et al. Unplanned readmissions of patients with congestive heart failure: do they reflect in-hospital quality of care or patient characteristics? *Am J Med* 2000;109:386–390.

18. Aghababian RV. Acutely decompensated heart failure: opportunities to improve care and outcomes in the emergency department. *Rev Cardiovascular Med* 2002;3[Suppl 4]:S3–9.

19. Kleinpell R, Gawlinski A. Assessing outcomes in advanced practice nursing practice. *AACN Clin Issues* 2005;16:43–57.

20. Butler J, Arbogast PG, Daugherty J, et al. Outpatient utilization of angiotensin-converting enzyme inhibitors among heart failure patients after hospital discharge. *J Am Coll Cardiol* 2004;43:2036–2043.

21. Hardin S, Hussey L. AACN synergy model for patient care: case study of a CHF patient. *Crit Care Nurse* 2003;23:73–76.

22. Barth V. A nurse managed discharge program for congestive heart failure patients: outcomes and costs. *Home Health Care Manage Pract* 2001;13:436–443.

23. Cline CMF, et al. Cost effective management programme for heart failure reduces hospitalization. *Heart* 1998;80:442–446.

24. Roe-Prior P. Variables predictive of poor post-discharge outcomes for hospitalized elders in heart failure. *West J Nurs Res* 2004;26:533–546.

25. Bosson O. The role of the heart failure specialist nurse. *Chest Medicine On-Line 2002.* Available at http://www.priory.com (accessed Sept. 24, 2005).

26. Koelling TM, Johnson ML, Cody RJ, et al. Discharge education improves clinical outcomes in patients with chronic heart failure. *Circulation* 2005;111:179–185.

27. Jaarsma T. Inter-professional team approach to patients with heart failure. *Heart* 2005;91:832–838.

28. Krumholz HM, Amatruda J, Smith GL, et al. Randomized trial of education and support intervention to prevent readmission of patient with heart failure. *J Am Coll Cardiol* 2002;39:83–89.

29. Hussey LC, et al. Outpatient costs of medications for patients with chronic heart failure. *Am J Crit Care* 2002;11:474–478.

30. Anthony MK, Hudson-Barr D. A patient-centered model of care for hospital discharge. *Clin Nurs Res* 2004;13:117–136.

31. Hanyu N, Nauman D, Burgess D, et al. Factors influencing knowledge of and adherence to self-care among patients with heart failure. *Arch Intern Med* 1999;159:1613–1619.

32. West JA, Miller NH, Parker KM, et al. A comprehensive management system for heart failure improves clinical outcomes and reduces medical resource utilization. *Am J Cardiol* 1997;79:58–63.

33. Dalton CC, Gottlieb LN. The concept of readiness to change. *J Adv Nurs* 2003; 42:108–117.

34. Morrow DG, Weiner M, Young J, et al. Improving medication knowledge among older adults with heart failure: a patient centered approach to instruction design. *Gerontologist* 2005;45:545–553.

35. Schneider JK, Hornberger S, Booker J, et al. A medication discharge planning program: measuring the effects on readmission. *Clin Nurs Res* 1993;2:41–53.

36. Cesta TG, Tahan HA. *The case managers survival guide: winning strategies for clinical practice,* 2nd ed. St. Louis: Mosby, 2003.

37. Kasper EK, Gerstenblith G, Hefter G, et al. A randomized trial of the efficacy of multidisciplinary care in heart failure outpatients at high risk of hospital readmission. *J Am Coll Cardiol* 2002;39:471–480.

38. Hunt SA, Abraham WT, Chin MH, et al. ACC/AHA 2005 guideline update for the diagnosis and management of chronic heart failure in the adult-summary article: a report of the American College of Cardiology/American Heart Association Task Force on Practice Guidelines (Writing Committee to Update the 2001 Guidelines for the Evaluation and Management of Heart Failure). *Circulation* 2005;112:e154–e235.

12

CHRONIC HEART FAILURE MANAGEMENT: DRUGS RECOMMENDED FOR ROUTINE USE

Robert J. Stomel and Majid J. Qazi

Multiple studies have established that chronic stable heart failure patients should be on four types of medications: (a) a diuretic, (b) angiotensin-converting enzyme inhibitor (ACEI), (c) a beta-blocker, and (d) digitalis.[1] Diuretics improve symptoms of heart failure patients by acutely removing fluid from the lung and by decreasing left ventricular filling pressures. Chronically, diuretics will decrease left ventricular wall stress and help slow the progression of remodeling. ACEIs result in left ventricular remodeling, which can ultimately reverse left ventricular dysfunction. Beta-blockers improve heart failure survival,[2] and digoxin can cause a decrease in heart failure hospitalizations.[3]

ANGIOTENSIN-CONVERTING ENZYME INHIBITORS

ACEIs are the foundation of heart failure therapy. They have beneficial effects for both the symptomatic and asymptomatic patient with left ventricular dysfunction. They reduce mortality,[4] decrease hospitalizations, enhance clinical status, and improve overall feeling of well-being.[5,6] Their mechanism and action are multifactorial. Initially, they were used as afterload-reducing agents. It is now known that ACEIs reduce myocardial volume and improve ejection fraction by left ventricular remodeling.[7,8] They also reduce norepinephrine levels[9] and enhance the action of kinins.[10] ACEIs should be started at a low dose and titrated upward as tolerated. Aspirin therapy may attenuate the benefit of ACEIs by blocking the effects of kinin-mediated prostaglandin synthesis.[11] ACEI use is contraindicated in patients with angioedema and anuric renal failure. They must be used very cautiously in patients who are hypotensive (blood pressure <80 mm Hg), hyponatremic, or hyperkalemic or whose serum creatinine is greater than 3.0 µg/mL.[12]

128

BETA-ADRENERGIC RECEPTOR BLOCKERS

Beta-blockers are now included as first-line therapy in all patients with mild to moderate heart failure. These patients maintain an overstimulated sympathetic nervous system, resulting in high levels of circulating serum norepinephrine. Chronic stimulation results in myocyte necrosis, peripheral vasoconstriction,[13] cardiac hypertrophy, left ventricular dysfunction, and ventricular arrhythmias. These deleterious effects ultimately result in an increase in cardiac death. Beta-blockers produce a significant dose-dependent mortality and morbidity benefit. They reduce the risk of rehospitalization and lower the instance of sudden cardiac death and death from progressive heart failure.[14,15]

Beta-blockers should be started in low doses and titrated upward slowly. Acute decompensation can occur when starting beta-blockers, so patients should be euvolemic and already on a stable dose of ACEI. Specific target doses are as follows: metoprolol CR/XL 200 mg daily, bisoprolol 5 mg daily, and carvedilol 25 mg twice a day.[16,17] Titration should be stopped if a patient's heart rate is less than 55 beats/minute or systolic blood pressure is less than 85 mm Hg. It may take up to 3 months to see a significant clinical response from beta-blocker therapy. Patients with clinically unstable heart failure are often dependent on adrenergic stimulation and can decompensate when started on beta-blockers. In patients hospitalized for decompensated heart failure, the posthospitalization goal should be to maintain or resume their previous beta-blocker dose. A withdrawal or reduction of beta-blocker therapy may result in increased mortality.

ANGIOTENSIN II RECEPTOR BLOCKERS

Currently, these agents are primarily used as alternatives to ACEIs in patients with heart failure who are intolerant to ACEIs. In this setting, they have been shown to be as effective as ACEIs in reducing mortality and morbidity.[18] There is somewhat conflicting evidence on the addition of angiotensin receptor blockers (ARBs) to ACEI therapy. However, recent trials suggest that this combination reduces cardiovascular deaths and heart failure admissions, including those being treated with beta-blockers.[19] It should be noted that the combination of ARBs and ACEIs increases the likelihood of hypotension and significant rise in serum creatinine.

HYDRALAZINE-ISOSORBIDE DINITRATE

Recent data indicate that the combination of hydralazine and isosorbide dinitrate may have a mortality benefit in black patients with class III or IV heart failure when added to standard heart failure therapy. Based on the results of the A-HeFT trial, the U.S. Food and Drug Administration (FDA) has approved the use of BiDil (a tablet containing 20 mg of the nitrate and

37.5 mg of hydralazine taken three times daily) for self-identified black patients with heart failure.[20] Additionally, patients unable to tolerate ACEIs or ARBs may realize a mortality reduction with the addition of the combination of hydralazine-isosorbide dinitrate.

DIURETICS

The first and most important goal in the treatment of acute decompensated heart failure is to relieve the symptoms of shortness of breath, coughing, and congestion from fluid overload. Loop diuretics (furosemide, bumetanide, and torsemide) are the only medications that achieve this goal. They are important in the treatment of acute decompensated heart failure and are necessary to prevent heart failure reoccurrence. They are a requirement for the successful integration of all other medications used for the treatment of heart failure. Furosemide, the most commonly used loop diuretic, unfortunately has variable absorption when taken orally. Torsemide is more consistent and can be substituted for furosemide if the patient is no longer obtaining an appropriate diuretic response. Diuretic resistance can also occur when a patient consumes large amounts of dietary sodium or develops prerenal azotemia. Nonsteroidal anti-inflammatory drugs (NSAIDs) can also block the effect of loop diuretics.[21] Complications of diuretics include intravascular volume depletion, arrhythmias, and renal insufficiency. Overdiuresis can result in a decrease in stroke volume, cardiac output, and left ventricular filling pressure. This can especially occur in patients with heart failure caused by diastolic dysfunction.

SPIRONOLACTONE

Patients with heart failure have increased activation of the renin-angiotensin-aldosterone system, resulting in high levels of circulating aldosterone. This potentiates heart failure through sympathetic activation and sodium retention. Aldosterone antagonists (spironolactone) should be considered for use in selected patients: those with New York Heart Association (NYHA) Class III/IV heart failure. A large multicenter study, Randomized Aldactone Evaluation Study (RALES), involving these patients demonstrated that the addition of spironolactone resulted in a 30% reduction in the risk of death (35% vs. 46%, p <.001).[22] These patients should be monitored closely for hyperkalemia. The medication should not be initiated if serum potassium levels are greater than 5.0 mg/dL or creatinine is greater than 2.5 mg/dL. For those intolerant to spironolactone, eplerenone may be used. Eplerenone is a selective aldosterone inhibitor with a significantly decreased incidence of the complications of gynecomastia and impotence. Careful monitoring and surveillance of laboratory studies is required while patients are on spironolactone, and doses of potassium supplementation may need to be decreased.

CARDIAC GLYCOSIDES

Cardiac glycosides (digoxin) inhibit Na^+/K^+ ATPase, which promotes Ca^{2+}/Na^+ exchange, producing a positive inotropic action. These drugs also reduce serum levels of circulating norepinephrine and return parasympathetic tone to heart failure patients.[23] In patients with mild to moderate heart failure, digoxin improves clinical symptoms and exercise tolerance and decreases hospitalizations. Unfortunately, it does not improve patient survival.[24] Digoxin is not indicated as a primary therapy for patients in acute decompensated heart failure. It is not necessary to use a loading dose in patients with heart failure, and serum digoxin levels are not particularly useful as a guide for adjusting digoxin dosage.[25] Most patients will respond to 0.125 mg of digoxin a day and there are no data to indicate improved effect on contractility with a larger dose. Digoxin is contraindicated in patients with sick sinus syndrome, second- and third-degree heart block, hypertrophic cardiomyopathy, Wolff-Parkinson-White syndrome, hypercalcemia, and hypokalemia.

SUMMARY

The seven golden rules of heart failure are as follows:

1. ACEIs are the cornerstone of chronic heart failure treatment. Start with a low dose and titrate to a moderate dose.
2. Aspirin and NSAIDs can block the favorable benefits of ACEIs.
3. Beta-blockers are a first-line therapy in heart failure treatment, but they should be started only after a patient is euvolemic and already on chronic ACEI therapy. Start with a low dose and titrate up slowly. Patients with stage 4 heart failure may be dependent on an adrenergic response and therefore can be intolerant to beta-blockers.
4. Overdiuresis can lead to hypotension and renal insufficiency. This may make heart failure worse, especially in patients with diastolic dysfunction.
5. Use spironolactone only in selected patients. Know which patient population was excluded in the RALES study.
6. There is no loading dose for digoxin, and serum levels are of little use.
7. Avoid antiarrhythmics, nonsteroidals, and calcium channel blockers.

REFERENCES

1. Packer M, Cohen JM, Abraham WT, et al. Consensus recommendation for the management of chronic heart failure. *Am J Cardiol* 1999;83:1A–38A.
2. Heidenreich PA, Lee TT, Massie BM. Effective beta blockade on mortality in patients with heart failure: a meta analysis of randomized clinical trials. *J Am Coll Cardiol* 1997; 30:27–34.
3. Digitalis Investigation Group: the effect of digoxin on mortality and morbidity in patients with heart failure. *N Engl J Med* 1997;336:525–533.
4. Effect of enalapril on survival in patients with reduced left ventricular ejection fractions and congestive heart failure. The SOLVD Investigators. *N Engl J Med* 1991;325:293–302.

5. A placebo controlled trial of captopril in refractory chronic congestive heart failure. Captopril Multi-Center Research Group. *J Am Coll Cardiol* 1983;2:755–763.

6. Erhardt L, MacClean A, Ilgenfritz J, et al. Fosinopril attenuates clinical deterioration and improves exercise tolerance in patients with heart failure. Fosinopril Efficacy/Safety Trial (FEST) Study Group. *Eur Heart J* 1995;16:182–189.

7. Greenberg B, Quinones MA, Koilpillai C, et al. Effects of long term enalapril on cardiac structure and function in patients with left ventricular dysfunction. *Circulation* 1995;91:2573–2581.

8. Constam MA, Rousseau MF, Kronenberw MW, et al. Effects of angiotensin converting enzyme inhibitor enalapril on the long term prognosis of left ventricular function in patients with heart failure. *Circulation* 1992;86:431–438.

9. Benedict C, Frances GS, Shelton B, et al. Effects of long term enalapril therapy on neurohormones in patients with left ventricular dysfunction. *Am J Cardiol* 1995;75:1151–1157.

10. Gainer JV, Morrow JD, Loveland A, et al. Effect of bradykinin-receptor blockade on the response of angiotensin converting enzyme inhibitor in normotensive and hypertensive subjects. *N Engl J Med* 1998;339:1285–1292.

11. Neward L, Khadra AS, Salem DN, et al. Antiplatelet agents in survival: a cohort analysis of the studies of left ventricular dysfunction (SOLVD) Trial. *J Am Cardiol* 1998;31:419–425.

12. Hunt SA, Baker DW, Chin MH, et al. ACC/AHA guidelines for the evaluation and management of chronic heart failure in the adult: executive summary: a report of the American College of Cardiology/American Heart Association Task Force on Practice Guidelines (Committee to Revise the 1995 Guidelines for the Evaluation and Management of Heart Failure). *J Am Coll Cardiol* 2001;38:2101–2113.

13. Smith KM, MacMillin JB, McGrath JC. Investigation of alpha one adrenoceptor subtypes mediating vasoconstriction in rabbit cutaneous resistance arteries. *Br J Pharmacol* 1997;122:825–832.

14. Parker M, Bristow MR, Cohen JN, et al. The effect of carvedilol on morbidity and mortality in patients with chronic heart failure. U.S. Carvedilol Heart Failure Study Group. *N Engl J Med* 1996;334:1349–1355.

15. Packer M, Coats AJ, Fowler MD, et al. Effects of carvedilol on survival in severe chronic heart failure. *N Engl J Med* 2001;344:1651–1658.

16. Packer M, Coats AJ, Fowler MB, et al. For the Carvedilol Prospective Randomized Cumulative Survival Study Group. Effect of carvedilol on survival in severe chronic heart failure. *N Engl J Med* 2001;334:1651–1658.

17. Dargie HJ. Effects of carvedilol on outcome after myocardial infarction in patients with left ventricular dysfunction: the CAPRICORN randomized trial. *Lancet* 2001;357:1385–1390.

18. McMurray JJ, Ostergren J, Swedberg K, et al. Effects of candesartan in patients with chronic heart failure and reduced left ventricular systolic function taking angiotensin-converting-enzyme inhibitors: the CHARM-Added trial. *Lancet* 2003;362:767–771.

19. Granger CB, McMurray JJ, Yusuf S, et al. Effects of candesartan in patients with chronic heart failure and reduced left-ventricular systolic function intolerant to angiotensin-converting-enzyme inhibitors: the CHARM-Alternative trial. *Lancet* 2003;362:772–776.

20. Taylor AL, Ziesche S, Yancy C, et al. Combination of isosorbide dinitrate and hydralazine in blacks with heart failure. *N Engl J Med* 2004;351:2049–2057.

21. Gottlieb SS, Robinson S, Krichten CM, Fisher NL. Renal response to indomethacin in congestive heart failure secondary to ischemic or idiopathic dilated cardiomyopathy. *Am J Cardiol* 1992;70:890–893.

22. RALES Study. Randomized Aldactone Evaluation Study. Investigators: Pitt B, Zanad F, Remme WJ, Cody R, Castaigne A, Perez A, et al. The effect of spironolactone on morbidity and mortality in patients with severe heart failure. *N Engl J Med* 1999;341:709–717.

23. Krum H, Bigger JT, Goldsmith RL, Packer M. Effect of long-term digoxin therapy to autonomic function in patients with chronic heart failure. *J Am Coll Cardiol* 1995; 25:289–294.

24. Digitalis Investigation Group. The effect of digoxin on mortality and morbidity in patients with heart failure. *N Engl J Med* 1997;336:525–533.

25. Hoeschen RJ, Cuddy TE. Dose-response relation between therapeutic levels of serum digoxin and systolic time intervals. *Am J Cardiol* 1975;35:469–472.

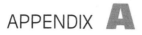

TREATMENT PATHWAYS AND ALGORITHMS

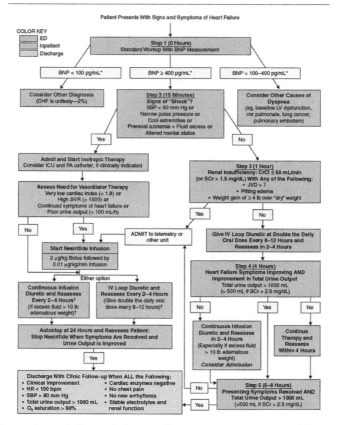

Algorithm for early goal-directed therapy for acute decompensated heart failure. ED, emergency department; BNP, B-type natriuretic peptide; CHF, congestive heart failure; ICU, intensive care unit; PA, pulmonary artery; SVR, systemic vascular resistance; HR, heart rate; SBP, systolic blood pressure; LV, left ventricular; CrCl, creatinine clearance; SCr, serum creatinine; JVD, jugular venous distention. *Clinical decisions should not be based solely on BNP level. BNP levels shown are for the Triage (Biosite) assay. †Consider decreasing dose of diuretic by 50% if receiving nesiritide. Adapted from Saltzberg MT. Beneficial Effects of Early Initiation of Vasoactive Agents in Patients With Acute Decompensated Heart Failure. *Rev Cardiovasc Med.* 2004;5(suppl 4):S17–S27.

Page available in full form on CD

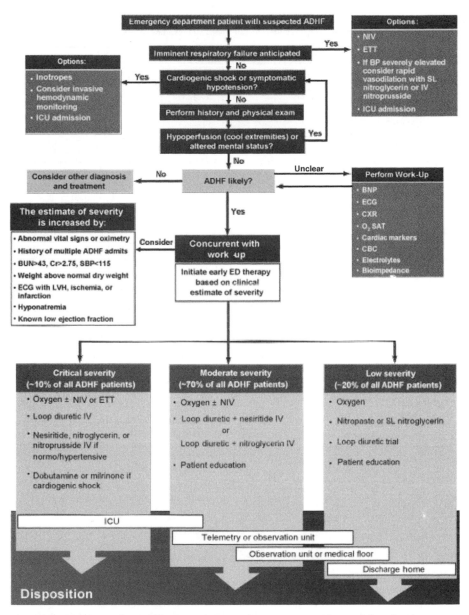

Algorithm for the early stabilization of acute decompensated heart failure in the emergency department. ADHF = acute decompensated heart failure; BNP = B-type natriuretic peptide; BUN = blood urea nitrogen; CBC = complete blood count; Cr = creatinine; CXR = chest radiograph; ECG = electrocardiogram; ETT = endotracheal tube; ICU = intensive care unit; LVH = left ventricular hypertrophy; NIV = non-invasive ventilation; O$_2$SAT = oxygen saturation; prn = as needed; SBP = systolic blood pressure; SL = sublingual.

Adapted from Peacock WF, Allegra J, Ander D, et al. Management of acutely decompensated heart failure in the emergency department. *CHF* 2003;9(suppl 1):3–18.

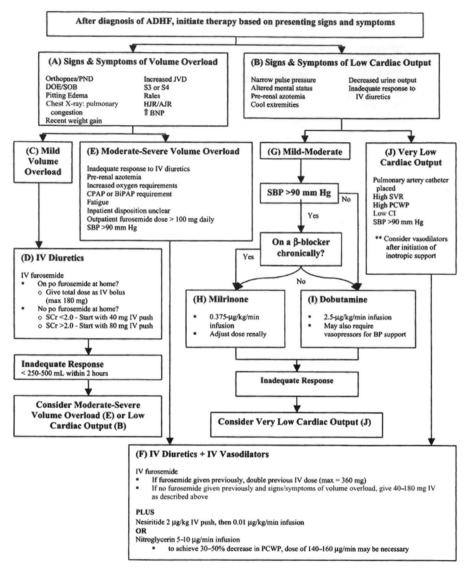

Acute decompensated heart failure (ADHF) treatment algorithm. AJR = abdominal jugular reflex; BiPAP = bilevel positive airway pressure; BNP = b-natriuretic peptide; CI = cardiac index; CPAP = continuous positive airway pressure; DOE = dyspnea on exertion; HJR = hepatojugular reflex; JVD = jugular venous distention; PCWP = pulmonary capillary wedge pressure; PND = paroxysmal nocturnal dyspnea; SBP = systolic blood pressure; SCr = serum creatinine; SOB = shortness of breath; SVR = systemic vascular resistance.

Adapted from DiDomenico RJ, Park HY, Southworth MR, et al. Guidelines for acute decompensated heart failure treatment. *Ann Pharmacother.* 2004;38:649–660.

Emergency Medicine Heart Failure Algorithm

Stat ED-HF Consensus Panel

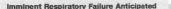

Emergency Department Patient with Suspected
Acutely Decompensated Heart Failure

Imminent Respiratory Failure Anticipated — YES →

Options
- BiPAP/CPAP Trial
- Endotracheal Intubation
- If BP Elevated, Consider Rapid Vasodilation with Nitroglycerin, Nesiritide or Nitroprusside
- ICU Admission

NO ↓

YES ← Cardiogenic Shock or Symptomatic Hypotension?

Options
- Inotropes
- Consider Hemodynamic Monitoring
- ICU Admission

NO ↓

Perform History and Physical Exam

↓

Hypoperfusion (cool extremities) or Altered Mental Status? — YES

NO ↓

Perform Workup
- BNP
- ECG
- CXR
- O2 SAT
- Cardiac Markers
- CBC
- Electrolytes

Consider Other Diagnosis and Treatment ← NO — Decompensated Heart Failure Likely? — UNSURE

YES ↓

Concurrent with Workup
Initiate Early ED Therapy Based on Clinical Estimate of Severity

↓

Critical Severity (~10% of all HF patients)	**Moderate Severity** (~80% of all HF patients)	**Low Severity** (~10% of all HF patients)
• Oxygen • Loop Diuretic • Nesiritide, Nitroglycerin or Nitroprusside	• Oxygen • Loop Diuretic • Nesiritide • Nitropaste or SL Nitroglycerin PRN • Patient Education	• Oxygen • Nitropaste or SL Nitroglycerin PRN • Loop Diuretic Trial • Patient Education

Disposition

ICU

Telemetry or Observation Unit

Observation Unit or Medical Floor

Discharge Home

The Estimate of Severity Is Increased by:
- Abnormal Vital Signs or Oximetry
- History of Multiple HF Admits
- BUN >43 mg/dL
- SBP <115 mm Hg
- Creatinine >2.75 mg/dL
- Weight Above Normal Dry Weight
- ECG with LVH, Elevated BP
- ↑BUN, ↑Creatinine
- Known Low Ejection Fraction
- Poor Response to Therapy

Page available in full form on CD

ADHERE® Registry Heart Failure Critical Pathway

**Dyspnea, Orthopnea, Edema
Suspicion of Heart Failure**

History, Physical Exam
Considerations: Hx HF, Hx Chest Pain, CAD, DM, HTN, Infection, Anemia

Useful Findings:
Elevated Jugular Venous Pressure
An S3 and/or Mitral Regurgitation Murmur
Peripheral Edema

ECG: Evaluate for ACS, Ischemia, Arrhythmias

Helpful Diagnostic Findings:
CXR: CHF and/or Cardiomegaly
BNP >100 pg/mL

**Establish Diagnosis
Determine Hemodynamic Status:
Shock/Hypoperfusion vs Congestion**

Shock/Hypoperfusion
SBP <80 mm Hg, AMS,
Cool Extremities

Congestion
SBP ≥90 mm Hg, Dyspnea at Rest or
Min Exertion, Orthopnea, Edema

Initial Management:
Single Agent or Combination of Inotropes
Single Agent or Combination of Pressors
Supplemental Oxygen
Hemodynamic Monitoring in CCU/ICU
Mechanical Support

Initial Management:
IV Loop Diuretics
IV Nesiritide
Supplemental Oxygen, if indicated
Telemetry or Observation Unit

Once Compensated:
Optimize Oral Heart Failure Medications
(ACE Inhibitors, Beta-blockers, Aldosterone Antagonists)
Evaluate/Manage Comorbidities; Assess Sudden Death Risk
Optimize Heart Failure Patient Education
Optimize Discharge Planning and Follow-up Care

Discharge

This treatment algorithm represents only one approach to the management of patients with heart failure. It is provided solely as a guide, and the decision regarding the specific care of a particular patient must be made by, and is the responsibility of, the physician and patient in light of all the circumstances presented by that patient.

Adapted by The ADHERE Registry Scientific Advisory Committee and based on UCLA Medical Center's Heart Failure Critical Pathway.

PLEASE SEE FULL PRESCRIBING INFORMATION ON REVERSE.

Adhere

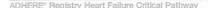

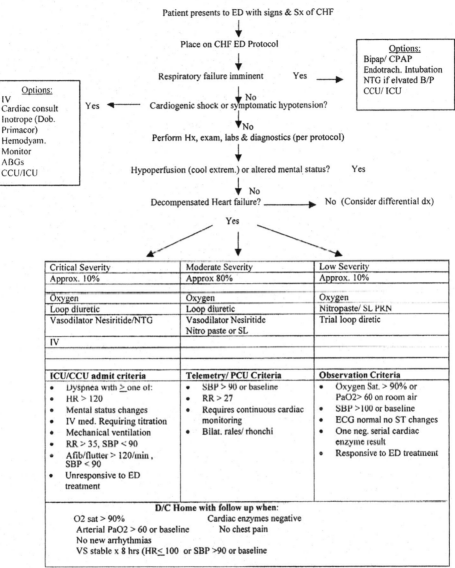

CHF Level of Care Algorithm
Florida Hospital Draft

Patient presents to ED with signs & Sx of CHF

Place on CHF ED Protocol

Respiratory failure imminent   Yes ⟶

Options:
Bipap/ CPAP
Endotrach. Intubation
NTG if elvated B/P
CCU/ ICU

No

Cardiogenic shock or symptomatic hypotension?   Yes ⟵

Options:
IV
Cardiac consult
Inotrope (Dob.
Primacor)
Hemodyam.
Monitor
ABGs
CCU/ICU

No

Perform Hx, exam, labs & diagnostics (per protocol)

Hypoperfusion (cool extrem.) or altered mental status?   Yes

No

Decompensated Heart failure? ⟶ No (Consider differential dx)

Yes

Critical Severity	Moderate Severity	Low Severity
Approx. 10%	Approx 80%	Approx. 10%
Oxygen	Oxygen	Oxygen
Loop diuretic	Loop diuretic	Nitropaste/ SL PRN
Vasodilator Nesiritide/NTG	Vasodilator Nesiritide Nitro paste or SL	Trial loop diretic
IV		
ICU/CCU admit criteria	**Telemetry/ PCU Criteria**	**Observation Criteria**
• Dyspnea with ≥ one of:	• SBP > 90 or baseline	• Oxygen Sat. > 90% or
• HR > 120	• RR > 27	PaO2> 60 on room air
• Mental status changes	• Requires continuous cardiac	• SBP >100 or baseline
• IV med. Requiring titration	monitoring	• ECG normal no ST changes
• Mechanical ventilation	• Bilat. rales/ rhonchi	• One neg. serial cardiac
• RR > 35, SBP < 90		enzyme result
• Afib/flutter > 120/min ,		• Responsive to ED treatment
SBP < 90		
• Unresponsive to ED		
treatment		

D/C Home with follow up when:

O2 sat > 90%   Cardiac enzymes negative
Arterial PaO2 > 60 or baseline   No chest pain
No new arrhythmias
VS stable x 8 hrs (HR≤ 100 or SBP >90 or baseline

*Comorbidities may affect decision for level of care placement

CONGESTIVE HEART FAILURE
Physician Protocol Checklist
(not part of medical record)

I. *Inclusion Criteria*
  – Patients must fulfill two of the following major inclusion criteria OR one major with two minor inclusion criteria
  ☐ Major
  ☐ Paroxysmal nocturnal dyspnea
  ☐ Cardiomegaly exhibited on chest X-ray
  ☐ Pulmonary edema exhibited on chest X-ray
  ☐ Neck distension
  ☐ Rales
  ☐ S3 gallop
  ☐ Positive hepatojugular reflex
  ☐ Minor
  ☐ Pleural effusion exhibited on chest X-ray
  ☐ Extremity edema
  ☐ Hepatomegaly
  ☐ Night Cough
  ☐ Dyspnea on exertion
  ☐ Tachycardia
  ☐ BNP level greater than 100
  ☐ Anticipated length-of-stay in CHF Observational Unit greater than 12 hours and less than 23 hours
  ☐ Orders for admission to observation status signed, dated, and timed by attending physician
  ☐ Adequate follow-up and social support anticipated at time of discharge

II. *Exclusion Criteria*
  ☐ Troponin T >0.01 ng/ml or CKMB >5.8 ng/ml with a positive relative index
  ☐ Syncope
  ☐ Hypotension (systolic BP <90 mmHg)
  ☐ Hypoxia (O_2 saturation <90% on room air)
  ☐ Severe respiratory distress (respiration rate >40)
  ☐ Patient on dialysis
  ☐ Blood pressure greater than 220/110
  ☐ Temperature greater than 100.0
  ☐ Heart rate greater than 130
  ☐ Severe electrolyte imbalances
  ☐ New ischemic changes on EKG (ST segment elevation/depression or T wave inversion)
  ☐ Unstable vital signs, shock, or severe systemic illness
  ☐ Multiple or severe co-morbidities likely to significantly complicate disposition decision

Page available in full form on CD

☐ Patient considered high risk (not eligible for Observational Unit due to severity of condition)

III. *Responsibilities*
☐ Make sure that there is a copy of the ED treating physician's Rapid Diagnosis and Treatment Center (RDTC) admission summary
☐ Complete ECHO referral form (echocardiogram needs to be performed if not completed in the last 6 months)
☐ Complete rest SPECT scan referral form (if you order this as part of work-up)
☐ If the patient is enrolled in the RDTC Protocol and does NOT have a physician to follow them up, please page the CHF Nurse Practitioner's voice mail (584-0323) so that they may arrange follow up).
☐ Administer pneumococcal vaccine if applicable
   – Any patient with CHF who has not received a vaccine should receive it
   – If a CHF patient has already received the vaccine, they should get revaccinated if:
      ○ If they have received their first vaccination when they <65 years old
      ○ ≥ 5 years since their last vaccination

III. *Disposition Criteria*
   HOME
☐ Discharge criteria
   – Negative biomarkers of cardiac ischemia
   – Room air saturation of greater than 90%
   – Systolic BP >90 mmHg
   – HR <100 beats per minute
   – No significant electrolyte abnormalities
   – No new arrhythmias or ECG changes
   – Negative results on functional study for myocardial ischemia
☐ Negative provocative testing (rest SPECT scan)
☐ Echo performed
☐ Patient must be observed in the RDTC for three hours following discontinuation of Nesiritide drip
☐ Stable vital signs and symptomatic improvement
☐ Final BNP level drawn
☐ Follow up scheduled at the Heart Failure Clinic
☐ Consultation for discharge medication regime
   – Monday–Friday: Heart Failure nurse practitioner
   – Saturday and Sunday: Heart Failure attending
☐ Heart Failure attending contacted if there is a question concerning discharge vs admission.
☐ Completed CHF Observational Unit Discharge Dictation
☐ Discharge order signed, dated, and timed by attending physician

Page available in full form on CD

HOSPITALIZATION CRITERIA

☐ Discharge criteria
- Positive biomarkers of cardiac ischemia
- Room air saturation less than 90% after treatment
- Systolic BP <90 mmHg
- HR >100 beats per minute
- Significant electrolyte abnormalities
- New arrhythmias or ECG changes
- Positive results on functional study for myocardial ischemia

☐ Unstable vital signs

☐ Positive provocative testing

☐ Does not meet discharge criteria after 23 hours of treatment

☐ Any patient with new-onset CHF needs to be admitted regardless of response to therapy per agreement with cardiology (please indicate in discharge summary if patient had responded to therapy and could have been sent home had they not been "new-onset" CHF)

☐ At the discretion of the ED physician, primary physician, or consulting cardiologist

Observation Congestive Heart Failure Patient Pathway

This pathway is a guide of what generally occurs for patients with your same diagnosis. Your doctor and staff caring for your may alter this plan to meet your needs.

Date_____ Today's Blood Pressure_____ Today's Weight_____

Therapies	Day One
Diagnostic Tests	• A Variety of tests will be done to see how efficiently your heart is working. These may include: • Chest x-ray (picture of your heart and lungs.) This will show if there is fluid in your lungs. • EKG (Allows the physician to look at different areas of your heart.) • Echocardiogram (ultrasound of your heart.) • Multiple blood tests today. These are very important to help your physician find any problems that can occur when you have a fluid imbalance in your body. These problems can usually be corrected with medications. • Other tests may be needed and will be explained to you. • Blood will be drawn on admission and 2-3 more times in the next 24 hours.
Medications and IV's	• You will have an IV in your arm or hand. • You will receive medications to help the work load and improve the pumping action of your heart and to help you get rid of excess fluid. Your doctor, nurse, or pharmacist will discuss your specific medications with you. Ask any questions you may have.
Treatments	• You will probably need oxygen, the type will depend on how well you are breathing and how high your oxygen levels are. • A finger clip monitor will be used to measure your oxygen levels. Your oxygen amount will be adjusted and then removed as your progress. • The nurse will weigh you each day and measure the amount of fluid you take in and the amount you put out. This is very important to see how much fluid your medication is removing from your body. You will get medications that will cause you to urinate frequently. • Your nurse will measure your blood pressure, pulse, breathing and temperature frequently today. She/he will also listen to your heart and lungs for signs of progress. • You will be on a heart monitor.
Diet	• You will be on a no-added salt diet after your shortness of breath has improved. Salt causes your body to hold fluid. A salt substitute will be available if you need it. • Your fluid intake will need to be measured. • The amount of fluid you drink will be adjusted according to your needs.
Consults/ Therapies	• If you have special problems or conditions, your doctor may ask a specialist to see you.
Activity	• Your activity will be encouraged as you can tolerate it. • You should avoid becoming overtired. • A bedside commode will be provided for your comfort.
Education	• You need to know what is going on inside your body. You will be given a learning booklet. Please ask questions if you do not understand your plan of care. • Congestive heart failure is not a heart attack. It means that the heart is not pumping enough blood to adequately meet the needs of the body, leading to a build up of fluid. Your symptoms may include shortness of breath, sweating, decreased appetite and fatigue. Your nurse can discuss this more in depth with you.
Discharge Planning/ Outcomes	• By the end of the day today you should feel better. Try to sleep well tonight.

Pvchf/h/mgdcr/dm/8/10/98, rev06/24/05

Observation Congestive Heart Failure Patient Pathway

Date_____   **Today's Blood Pressure**_____   **Today's Weight**_____

Therapies	Day Two
Diagnostic Tests	• More blood tests as well as another x-ray will be done to measure your heart's progress. • Your blood work will be used as a guide when adjusting medication.
Medications and IV's	• Medications may be changed from IV to pill form today. • Plan your medication schedule for when you go home. Your nurse or pharmacist can help you work this out.
Treatments	• Your oxygen should be stopped today if you can walk in the hallways without trouble breathing. • Your heart will be continue to be monitored. • You will be weighed again, and your ankle swelling should be less than yesterday. You should continue this at home and notify your doctor if you gain 2 lbs or more. • Remember to continue to let your nurse know if you drink anything.
Diet	• Ask any questions or concerns you have about your diet. This is important. The fluid restriction your doctor ordered will also continue.
Consults/ Therapies	• Make sure you know which doctors you need to see after discharge and when.
Activity	• You should be able to walk in the hallways without trouble breathing.
Education	• Continue to review booklet and ask your nurse and physician any questions you need to ask. • Diet and weight management: you should know to weigh yourself every day. • Prevention • Signs and symptoms: you should know the worsening signs and symptoms of heart failure in order to report to your doctor immediately. • Disease process • Medications • Exercise
Discharge Planning/ Outcomes	• Your swelling should be gone. You should have lost the water weight and be breathing normally. • You should ask your nurse to help you identify your cardiac risk factors prior to discharge. • A social worker or continuing care nurse may be assigned to help you plan to go home. • You should be discharged from the hospital today.

Page available in full form on CD

MCP – Observation
Congestive Heart Failure

TRIGGERS:

Check the box to indicate the trigger has been completed, date & initial.

Phase One
☐ Height & Weight completed; message sent to Pharmacy: _____
☐ Cardiology consulted: _____
☐ BNP level done in ER: _____
☐ Cardiac biomarkers every 8 hrs x 3 ordered: _____
☐ Chest x-ray completed in ER: _____
☐ 2-D mode echo – LV function: _____
☐ 2 gm Na diet ordered: _____
☐ Fluid restrictions reviewed with patient / family: _____
☐ Ace inhibitor ordered: _____   ☐ Contraindicated because: _____
☐ Beta Blocker ordered: _____   ☐ Contraindicated because: _____
☐ Diuretic: _____
☐ K+ supplement: _____
☐ ASA: _____
☐ CHF teaching initiated: _____
☐ HF teaching booklet provided to patient/family: _____

Phase Two
☐ IV medications changed to oral: _____
☐ Ambulating pulse ox completed / recorded: _____
☐ Oxygen discontinued: _____
☐ Cardiac biomarkers reviewed / recorded: _____
☐ Repeat BNP completed: _____
☐ Repeat chest x-ray completed: _____
☐ CBC, lytes, mag / phos, BUN, creatine reviewed / recorded: _____
☐ RN instructed patient / family on low Na diet: _____
☐ Weight prior to discharge completed: _____
☐ Discharge plan confirmed: _____
☐ Nursing discharge form completed / signed: _____

Nurses Signatures					
Initials	*Full Signature*	*Initials*	*Full Signature*	*Initials*	*Full Signature*

8/3/2005

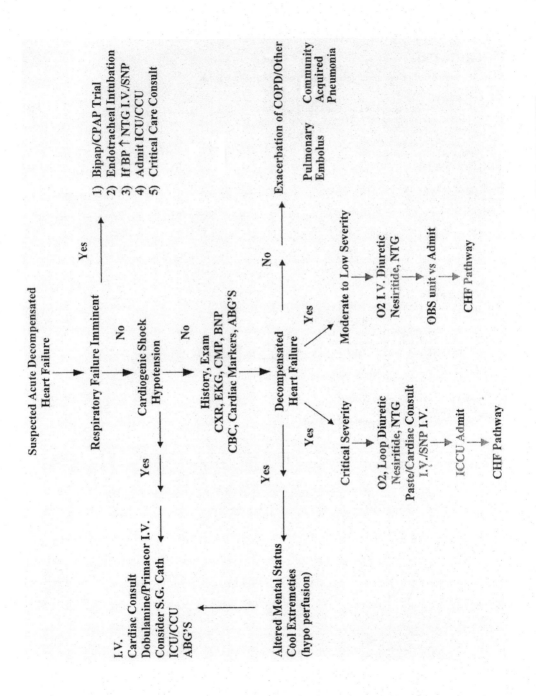

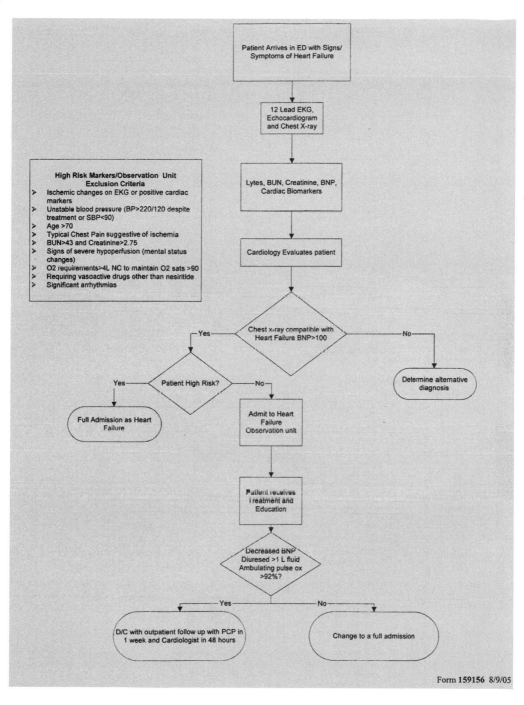

Patient Arrives in ED with Signs/
Symptoms of Heart Failure

12 Lead EKG,
Echocardiogram
and Chest X-ray

**High Risk Markers/Observation Unit
Exclusion Criteria**
➢ Ischemic changes on EKG or positive cardiac
  markers
➢ Unstable blood pressure (BP>220/120 despite
  treatment or SBP<90)
➢ Age >70
➢ Typical Chest Pain suggestive of ischemia
➢ BUN>43 and Creatinine>2.75
➢ Signs of severe hypoperfusion (mental status
  changes)
➢ O2 requirements>4L NC to maintain O2 sats >90
➢ Requiring vasoactive drugs other than nesiritide
➢ Significant arrhythmias

Lytes, BUN, Creatinine, BNP,
Cardiac Biomarkers

Cardiology Evaluates patient

Chest x-ray compatible with
Heart Failure BNP>100

—Yes— —No—

Determine alternative
diagnosis

Patient High Risk?

Yes— —No—

Full Admission as Heart
Failure

Admit to Heart
Failure
Observation unit

Patient receives
Treatment and
Education

Decreased BNP
Diuresed >1 L fluid
Ambulating pulse ox
>92%?

—Yes— —No—

D/C with outpatient follow up with PCP in
1 week and Cardiologist in 48 hours

Change to a full admission

Form **159156** 8/9/05

Page available in full form on CD

APPENDIX B

E.D. HEART FAILURE ORDERS

Instructions for inserting logos are available on the accompanying CD and in the back of this binder

1. DATE AND TIME ORDERS
2. CHECK ALL APPROPRIATE ORDERS

Emergency Medicine Heart Failure Orders

Emergency Medicine Physician: _____ Pager: _____

Primary Physician/Cardiologist: _____ Pager: _____

Etiology: _____ NYHA Class: _____ LVEF (if known): _____

DATE:

TIME:

Admit to: ☐ EMC ☐ EMC Observation Unit

MONITORING	☐ Cardiac monitoring
	☐ Pulse oximetry
	☐ Invasive lines:
VITAL SIGNS	☐ Per unit routine ☐ Other:
	☐ Call attending MD for an SBP >150, SBP <80 mm Hg, HR >100, HR <50, RR >24, or RR <8
CHARTING	☐ Obtain old records (chart, radiology)
ALLERGIES	☐ NKDA ☐ Allergy:
ACTIVITY	☐ Bed rest
	☐ Out of bed with assistance
FOLEY	☐ If patient is unable to void, place Foley catheter
IVs	☐ Initiate _____ peripheral IVs with _____ and draw blood
	☐ Heplock with 3 cc normal saline flush q 12 hours
	☐ Other:
I/O and WEIGHT	☐ Strict recording of Ins and Outs with running totals of urine output
	☐ Weight (chart results)
DIET	☐ NPO
	☐ 2 gram sodium diet
RESPIRATORY	☐ Oxygen ___L via nasal cannula (for CP, SOB, SaO2 <93%)
	☐ Oxygen ___% via face mask (for CP, SOB, SaO2 <93%)
	☐ CPAP at 5-7.5 cm H2O, oxygen bleed in to keep sats ≥ ____%
	☐ BiPAP at 10/5, oxygen bleed in to keep sats ≥ ____%
	☐ Ventilator settings (if intubated):
LABORATORIES	☐ CBC with differential and platelets
	☐ Electrolytes, BUN, creatinine, glucose
	☐ CPK total and MB NOW and q 8 hours x 3 or ☐ at _____
	☐ Cardiac troponin NOW and 6 hours or ☐ at _____
	☐ INR and ☐ PTT (if indicated)
	☐ BNP (if indicated)
	☐ Liver function tests (if indicated)
	☐ Cardiovascular lipid panel (if indicated)
	☐ Digoxin level (if patient receiving digoxin)
	☐ RUA
	☐ Others:
TESTING	☐ EKG
	☐ Chest x-ray (PA and lateral)
	☐ Arterial blood gas
	☐ Echocardiogram (portable)
	☐ Others:

148

Page available in full form on CD

MEDICATIONS

IV MEDICATIONS

Diuretics

☐ Furosemide _____ IVP and/or by   ☐ Continuous infusion at _____ mg/hr

☐ Bumetanide_____ IVP and/or by   ☐ Continuous infusion at _____ mg/hr

☐ KCL 40 mEq/250 D5W IVPB over 4 hours

Intravenous Vasodilators/Natriuretic Peptides

☐ Nesiritide 2 μg /kg IV bolus and then 0.01 μg /kg/min (hold for SBP <80 mm Hg)

Pressor Agent

☐ Dopamine 400 mg/250 mL D5W at _____ μg /kg/min IV drip

Adjuncts

☐ Nitroglycerin 0.4 mg SL q 5 min up to 4 times

☐ Morphine sulfate 2 mg IVP prn pain, anxiety, MR x 1 in 15 mins

ORAL MEDICATIONS

☐ Aspirin 325 mg PO first dose NOW and qd or

☐ Clopidogrel 300 mg PO NOW and 75 mg PO qd

☐ ACE inhibitor _____ mg PO _____ (hold for SBP <80 mm Hg)

☐ Beta-blocker _____ mg PO _____ (hold for SBP <80 mm Hg, should not be newly initiated for HF until patient is stable and no longer significantly volume-overloaded)

☐ Spironolactone _____ mg PO qd (use with caution if Cr >2.5, closely monitor K+)

☐ Furosemide_____ mg PO _____

☐ KCL _____ mEq _____

☐ Digoxin _____ mg PO qd

☐ Nitrate _____ mg PO _____ (hold for SBP <80 mm Hg)

☐ Statin _____ mg PO _____

☐ Warfarin _____ mg PO _____

☐ _____

☐ _____

☐ _____

☐ _____

☐ _____

☐ _____

DVT PROPHYLAXIS OR ANTICOAGULATION

☐ Enoxaparin _____ mg SQ _____

☐ Heparin 5000 mg SQ bid

☐ IV heparin protocol

PRN MEDICATIONS

☐ Acetaminophen 650 mg PO q 4 hours prn pain

☐ Oxycodone 5 mg/acetaminophen 325 mg (Percocet®) 2 tabs PO q 4 hours prn pain

☐ Morphine sulfate _____ mg IVP q 2 hours prn severe pain

☐ Diazepam (Valium®) 2 mg IVP q 4 hours prn for back pain or anxiety

☐ Maalox® Plus ES 15 mL PO qid prn gas or GI upset

☐ Prochlorperazine (Compazine®) 5 mg IV x 1 for vomiting. May repeat x 1 in 30 mins

☐ Nitroglycerin 0.4 mg SL q 5 min x 3 doses prn chest pain. Call MD/NP

☐ Serax 15 mg PO q hs prn insomnia. May repeat x 1 prn

☐ _____

☐ _____

MD Signature: _____   RN Signature: _____

Adhere®

Emergency Medicine Heart Failure Orders

Page available in full form on CD

1. DATE AND TIME ORDERS
2. CHECK ALL APPROPRIATE ORDERS

Heart Failure Admission Orders

Attending Physician: _____ Pager: _____

Consulting Cardiologist: _____ Pager: _____

Etiology: _____ NYHA Class: _____ LVEF (if known): _____

DATE:

TIME:

ORDER:
Admit to ☐ CCU   ☐ Telemetry   ☐ General Medical Floor   SERVICE: _____

DIET	☐ 2 gram sodium diet ☐ Other: ☐ 1800 cc fluid restriction ☐ Other:
VITAL SIGNS	☐ Per unit routine ☐ Other: _____ ☐ Call attending MD for an SBP >150, SBP <80 mm Hg, HR >100, HR <50, RR >24, or RR <8
ALLERGIES	☐ NKDA ☐ Allergy:
ACTIVITY	☐ Bed rest with commode privileges ☐ Out of bed with assistance ☐ Ambulation
FOLEY	☐ If patient is unable to void, place Foley catheter
IVs	☐ Heplock with 3 cc normal saline flush q 12 hours ☐ Other:
I/O and WEIGHT	☐ Strict recording of Ins and Outs with running totals of urine output ☐ Daily weights (chart results)
MONITORING	☐ Cardiac monitoring ☐ Pulse oximetry ☐ Lines:
RESPIRATORY	☐ Oxygen ___L via nasal cannula (for CP, SOB, SaO2 <93%) ☐ Oxygen ___% via face mask (for CP, SOB, SaO2 <93%) ☐ CPAP at 5-7.5 cm H2O, oxygen bleed in to keep sats ≥ _____% ☐ BiPAP at 10/5, oxygen bleed in to keep sats ≥ _____% ☐ Ventilator settings (if intubated):
LABORATORIES	☐ CBC with differential and platelets ☐ Electrolytes, BUN, creatinine, glucose ☐ CPK total and MB NOW and q 8 hours x 3 or ☐ at _____ ☐ Cardiac troponin NOW and 6 hours or ☐ at _____ ☐ INR and ☐ PTT (if indicated) ☐ BNP (if indicated) ☐ Liver function tests (if indicated) ☐ Cardiovascular lipid panel (if indicated) ☐ Digoxin level (if patient receiving digoxin) ☐ Others:
TESTING	☐ EKG ☐ Chest x-ray (PA and lateral) ☐ Arterial blood gas ☐ Echocardiogram ☐ Others:

Page available in full form on CD

MEDICATIONS	**IV MEDICATIONS**

Diuretics

☐ Furosemide _____ IVP and/or by   ☐ Continuous infusion at _____ mg/hr

☐ Bumetanide _____ IVP and/or by   ☐ Continuous infusion at _____ mg/hr

☐ KCL 40 mEq/250 D5W IVPB over 4 hours

Intravenous Vasodilators/Natriuretic Peptides

☐ Nesiritide 2 µg /kg IV bolus and then 0.01 µg /kg/min (hold for SBP <80 mm Hg)

Pressor Agent (titrate to _____)

☐ Dopamine 400 mg/250 mL D5W at _____ µg /kg/min IV drip

How was dopamine selected as the first-line pressor? _____
_____

ORAL MEDICATIONS

☐ Aspirin 325 mg PO first dose NOW and qd or

☐ Clopidogrel 300 mg PO NOW and 75 mg PO qd

☐ ACE inhibitor _____ mg PO_____ (hold for SBP <80 mm Hg, closely monitor K+)

☐ Beta-blocker _____ mg PO_____ (hold for SBP <80 mm Hg, should not be newly initiated for HF until patient is stable
  and no longer significantly volume-overloaded)

☐ Spironolactone _____ mg PO qd (use with caution if Cr >2.5, closely monitor K+)

☐ Furosemide _____ mg PO_____

☐ KCL_____ mEq ____

☐ Digoxin _____ mg PO qd

☐ Nitrate_____ mg PO_____ (hold for SBP <80 mm Hg)

☐ Statin _____ mg PO_____

☐ Warfarin _____ mg PO_____

☐ _____

☐ _____

☐ _____

☐ _____

☐ _____

☐ _____

DVT PROPHYLAXIS OR ANTICOAGULATION

☐ Enoxaparin _____ mg SQ _____

☐ Heparin 5000 mg SQ bid

☐ IV heparin protocol

PRN MEDICATIONS

☐ Acetaminophen 650 mg PO q 4 hours prn pain

☐ Oxycodone 5 mg/acetaminophen 325 mg (Percocet®) 2 tabs PO q 4 hours prn pain

☐ Morphine sulfate _____ mg IVP q 2 hours prn severe pain

☐ Diazepam (Valium®) 2 mg IVP q 4 hours prn for back pain or anxiety

☐ Maalox® Plus ES 15 mL PO qid prn gas or GI upset

☐ Prochlorperazine (Compazine®) 5 mg IV x 1 for vomiting. May repeat x 1 in 30 mins

☐ Nitroglycerin 0.4 mg SL q 5 min x 3 doses prn chest pain. Call MD/NP

☐ Serax 15 mg PO q hs prn insomnia. May repeat x 1 prn

☐ _____

☐ _____

PROTOCOLS	☐ Heart Failure Patient Education and Documentation

☐ Implement Discharge Teaching Protocol

☐ Nutrition Consultation and Counseling

☐ Smoking Cessation Counseling

☐ Cardiac Rehabilitation Assessment and Referral

MD Signature: _____   RN Signature: _____

*This sample template form is provided only as an example. You are solely responsible for determining
the appropriateness of its use and the content of any form that you develop from it.*

*Adapted by The ADHERE Registry Scientific Advisory Committee and based on
UCLA Medical Center's Heart Failure Admission Orders.*

Adhere®

Heart Failure Admission Orders

Evidence Based Practice- Heart Failure
EMERGENCY DEPARTMENT ORDERS

959-1618

DATE	TIME WRITTEN	NOTE: ORDERS MUST BE REVIEWED AND AUTHENTICATED BY RESPONSIBLE PHYSICIAN. Guidelines are not a substitute for the experience and judgment of a physician and are developed to enhance the physician's ability to practice evidence based medicine.
		1. Primary Diagnosis: Acute Decompensated CHF
		2. Check Oxygen Saturation, Initiate FH oxygen protocol, Continuous cardiac monitoring
		3. Intravenous access: Saline lock
		4. Labs: (If not already done) Comprehensive metabolic panel, Hemogram with platelets and differential, PT/INR, PTT
		Magnesium, Calcium, Phosphorus, B type natriuretic peptide (BNP) if not on nesiritide
		CPK-MB now, Troponin I now, Digoxin level (if on outpatient Digoxin)
		5. Testing (if not already done):
		12-Lead EKG
		Chest X-ray: ☐ PA & LAT ☐ Portable
		☐ 2-D Echo to be read by physician:
		6. Weigh patient (in ED if possible) Record all Intake and output ☐ Foley catheter
		Medications:
		7. ☐ ASA enteric coated 325milligrams by mouth ☐ ASA enteric coated 81milligrams by mouth
		8. **Diuretic:**
		☐ If not on Furosemide outpatient, give Furosemide 40 milligrams intravenous, times one dose.
		☐ If on Furosemide outpatient, give 24 hour home dose _____ milligrams, times one dose. Suggested Max dose 80mg
		☐ Other diuretic:
		Assess response to diuretic in 2 hours. If urine output is less than 1000 milliliters with normal renal function or less than 500 milliliters with renal insufficiency, consider Nesiritide (Natrecor) therapy.
		9. **I.V. Vasodilators: Hold if systolic blood pressure is less than:**
		☐ Nesiritide (Natrecor) Systolic blood pressure greater than 90 use standing order #959 - 1488
		☐ Nitroglycerin 50milligrams per 250 milliliters Dextrose 5% water intravenous at: _____ micrograms per minute
		(5 to 50 micrograms per minute.
		10. **Nitrates: Hold if systolic blood pressure is less than:**
		☐ Nitroglycerin paste: _____ inches topically every 12 hours
		11. **Inotropes: Hold if systolic blood pressure is less than:**
		☐ Milrinone 20milligrams per 100 milliliters Dextrose 5% water (200 micrograms per milliliters): _____ micrograms per
		kilogram per minute (0.375 to 0.75 micrograms per kilogram per minute).
		☐ Dobutamine 500milligrams per 250 milliliters Dextrose 5% water (2000 micrograms per milliliter) intravenous
		at: _____ micrograms per kilogram minute (2.5 to 20 micrograms per kilogram per minute).
		12. **Electrolyte Replacement:**
		☐ Potassium Chloride Protocol (#959-1295) ☐ Magnesium Protocol (#959-1494)

PHYSICIAN SIGNATURE

ALLERGIES: DIAGNOSIS: HEIGHT: WEIGHT:

FLORIDA HOSPITAL

EVIDENCE-BASED PRACTICE
A PASSION for EXCELLENCE

Evidence Based Practice
Heart Failure ED Orders
     (7/25/05) R- POD

Page available in full form on CD

| 959-1350 | **Heart Failure Admission Orders- Evidence Based Practice** | Page 1 of 2 |

DATE	TIME WRITTEN	
		NOTE: ORDERS MUST BE REVIEWED AND AUTHENTICATED BY RESPONSIBLE PHYSICIAN. Guidelines are not a substitute for the experience and judgment of a physician and are developed to enhance the physician's ability to practice evidence based medicine.
		ADMIT TO: ☐ Inpatient status **PLACE IN:** ☐ Outpatient/Observation status
		1. **Admit to:** ☐ PCU ☐ CCU/ICU Admitting Physician: Consult:
		2. **Diagnosis:** Congestive Heart Failure **Secondary diagnoses:**
		3. **Consult:** Case management, Cardiac Rehabilitation and Dietary. ☐ Physical Therapy Consult
		4. Left Ventricular Ejection Fraction less than 40%: ☐ Yes ☐ No ☐ Unknown
		5. Old Charts to Unit / include Cardiac Echo report if previously done
		6. **Intravenous Access:** Saline Lock with standard flush
		7. Strict Intake and Output. Weight on admission and daily using same scale.
		8. Vital Signs and Oxygen saturation per unit routine ☐ every hours.
		9. **Fluid restriction:** 2 liters per 24 hours ☐ Other: milliliters per day
		12. **Diet:** 2 gram Sodium Cardiac diet, no concentrated sweets if patient diabetic ☐ Other:
		13. ☐Oxygen: liter per minute nasal cannula per protocol ☐ Other: ☐ ABG
		14. **Labs:** (if not done in Emergency Department)
		Comprehensive metabolic panel, Hemogram with platelets, Magnesium, Fasting Lipid Panel in morning, Digoxin level (if on Digoxin)
		CPK-MB only every 4 hours X 3, Troponin I NOW and in 12 hours, B-type natriuretic peptic (BNP) (if not on Natrecor)
		Basic metabolic panel every morning X 3 days, Magnesium every morning X 3 days
		15. **Diagnostic Testing:** (if not done in Emergency Department)
		Chest x-ray: ☐ Portable ☐ PA/ and LAT ☐ 2-D Echo to be read by :
		EKG (if not done in ED)
		15. **Activity:**
		☐Bed Rest ☐ Bathroom Privileges With Assistance ☐ Up as desired, freely
		16. **Education:**
		A. Heart failure teaching: "CHF Discharge Care" via Micromedex Care notes/ HF packet
		B. Smoking cessation (for patients who have smoked within last 12 months) via Micromedex Care Notes
		Medications
		20. **Intravenous Vasodilators:**
		☐ Nesiritide (Natrecor) if systolic blood pressure greater than 90 (Use standing order #959-1488)
		☐ Nitroglycerin 50 milligrams per 250 milliliters Dextrose 5% in water (200 micrograms per milliliter) intravenously, micrograms per minute
		(5-50micrograms per minute)
		21. **Inotropes:**
		☐ Milrinone 20 milligrams/100 milliliter Dextrose 5% in Water(200 micrograms/milliliter) intravenously at micrograms/kilograms/minute
		(0.375- 0.75 micrograms/kilogram/minute)
		☐ Dobutamine 500milligram/250milliliters Dextrose 5% in Water (2000micrograms/milliliter) intravenously at micrograms/kilograms/minute
		(2.5 – 20 micrograms/kilogram/minute)

FLORIDA HOSPITAL

A **EVIDENCE-BASED PRACTICE**
A JOURNEY TOWARD EXCELLENCE

Evidence Based Practice
HF ADMISSION ORDERS
(07/25/05) R POD

Page 1 of 2

| 959-1350 | Heart Failure Admission Orders- Evidence Based Practice | Page 2 of 2 |

22. Diuretics:

☐ furosemide (Lasix)   milligrams intravenously every   hours   **OR**   milligrams orally daily

☐ bumetanide (Bumex)   milligrams intravenously every   hours   **OR**   milligrams orally daily

☐ torsimide (Demadex)   milligrams intravenously every   hours   **OR**   milligrams orally daily

☐ metolazone (Zaroxolyn)   milligrams orally daily   ☐ Hydrochorathiazide   milligrams orally every   hours.

23. Electrolyte Replacement

☐ FH Potassium Protocol (#959-1295)

☐ FH Magnesium Protocol (#959-1494)   ☐ Other:

24. ACE Inhibitors: Contraindication: **Hold for systolic blood pressure less than:**

☐ captopril (Capoten)   milligrams orally every   hours.

☐ ramipril (Altace)   milligrams orally daily.

☐ lisinopril (Zestril)   milligrams orally daily.

☐ enalapril (Vasotec)   milligrams orally every   hours.

25. Angiotensin II Receptor Antagonist: Contraindication: **Hold for systolic blood pressure less than:**

☐ valsartan (Diovan)   milligrams orally every 12 hours

☐ losartan (Cozaar)   milligrams orally daily

26. Beta Blockers: Contraindication: **Hold for systolic blood pressure less than:**

☐ carvedilol (Coreg)   milligrams orally every 12 hours, with meals.

☐ metoprolol (Lopressor)   milligrams every   hours.

27. Other

☐ spironalactone (Aldactone)   milligrams orally daily   ☐ eplerenone (Inspra)   milligrams orally daily

☐ digoxin (Lanoxin)   milligrams orally daily   ☐ hydralazine (Apresoline)   milligrams orally every 8 hours

☐ Aspirin enteric coated 325 milligrams orally daily   ☐ Aspirin enteric coated 81 milligrams orally daily

28. Nitrates:

Nitroglycerin 0.4 mg sublingual as needed for chest pain/angina

☐ isosorbide mononitrate (Imdur)   milligrams orally every   hours.

☐ Nitroglycerin Paste   inches topically every 12 hours   ☐ Nitroglycerin patch   milligrams/hour topically, daily. Remove at bedtime

29. DVT Prophylaxis: ☐ TED hose   ☐ Sequential Compression Device

☐ enoxaprin (Lovenox) 40 milligrams subcutaneously daily   ☐ Heparin 5000 units subcutaneously every 8 hours

30. Anticoagulation:

☐ warfarin (Coumadin)   milligrams orally daily   **Hold if INR greater than:**

☐ Draw PT/INR every day x   days

PHYSICIAN SIGNATURE:_____   DATE/TIME:_____

ALLERGIES: Patient Diagnosis: Height: Weight:

FLORIDA HOSPITAL

EVIDENCE-BASED PRACTICE
A JOURNEY TO EXCELLENCE

Evidence Based Practice
HF ADMISSION ORDERS
(07/25/05) R POD

Page 2 of 2

Page available in full form on CD

Congestive Heart Failure Order Set
For Acute Decompensated Congestive Heart Failure Patients
Emergency Department Order Sheet

Date   Time   Primary Diagnosis: Acute Decompensated Congestive Heart Failure
Secondary Diagnosis: _____
Vital signs q4h and as directed by medications (see individual medications)

❑ Labs: Basic metabolic panel, calcium, magnesium, phosphorus, CBC, PT/INR, PTT, BNP, CK, CK-MB, Troponin, O_2 saturation
❑ Digoxin level (if outpatient medication)
❑ Patient Weight: _____
❑ Ins and Outs
❑ 12 Lead ECG
❑ AP and lateral chest x-ray
❑ Foley catheter prn heavy diuresis
❑ Diet: <2.4g Na, low fat
❑ Fluid restriction: 1800 mL/24h; if Na <131 mg/dL, restrict fluid to 1500 mL/24h

Intravenous Furosemide
❑ If furosemide naïve, furosemide 40 mg IVP x 1 dose
❑ If on furosemide as outpatient
    Total daily dose as IV _____ mg: maximum 180 mg
    • Goal: >500 mL urine output within 2 hours for normal renal function
      >250 mL urine output within 2 hours if renal insufficiency
    • If goal urine output not met within 2 hours, double the furosemide dose to a maximum of 360 mg IV
    • Monitor symptom relief, vital signs, BUN, SCr, electrolytes

Nesiritide
❑ 2 µg IV push followed by 0.01 µg/kg/min IV infusion
❑ If symptomatic hypotention during infusion, discontinue nesiritide
    • Monitor symptom relief, vital signs q15m × 1 hour, then q30min × 1 hour, then q4h, urine output, electrolytes, BUN, SCr, magnesium, calcium, phosphorus
❑ If poor symptom relief or diuretic response ≥3 hours after nesiritide therapy initiation AND SBP ≥90 mm Hg, may consider titration of nesiritide
    • Nesiritide 1 µg/kg IVP and increase infusion by 0.005 µg/kg/min
    • May increase infusion rate q1h after first dosage, increase to a maximum dose of 0.03 µg/kg/min

Nitroglycerin 50 mg/250 mL
❑ 5 µg/min IV infusion; titrate dose q5min by 10–20 µg/min to achieve symptom relief
    • Monitor symptom relief, vital signs q15min until stable dose, then q30min × 1 hour, then q4h, ECG, urine output

Dobutamine 500 mg/250 mL
❑ 2.5 µg/kg/min IV infusion and titrate dose every 5 minutes to desired response to a maximum dose of 20 µg/kg/min
    • Monitor symptom relief, vital signs q15min until stable dose, then q30min × 1 hour, then q4h; ECG; urine output

Milrinone 20 mg/100 mL
❑ 0.375 µg/kg/min
    • Monitor symptom relief, vital signs q15min until stable dose, then q30min × 1 hour, then q4h; ECG; urine output

Page available in full form on CD

❏ Digoxin _____

Dose   Route   Frequency

❏ Lisinopril PO _____

Dose   Frequency

❏ Losartan PO _____

Dose   Frequency

❏ Metoprolol PO _____

Dose   Frequency

❏ Spironolactone PO _____

Dose   Frequency

Electrolyte Replacement

❏ Potassium

level (mEq/L)	IV dose (over 1 h)	PO dose	When to recheck potassium
3.7–3.9	20 mEq	40 mEq	12 hours or next morning
3.4–3.6	20 mEq × 2 doses	40 mEq × 2 doses	6 hours or next morning
3.0–3.3	20 mEq × 4 doses	40 mEq × 3 doses	4 hours after last dose
<3.0	20 mEq × 6 doses	Give IV only	1 hour after last dose

- If Clcr <30 mL/min, reduce dose by 50%

❏ Magnesium

level (mEq/L)	IV dose	PO dose (Mg oxide)	When to recheck magnesium
1.9	Give PO only	140 mg	Next morning
1.3–1.8	1 g $MgSO_4$ for every 0.1 below 1.9 (max 6 g)	Give IV only	Next morning
<1.3	8 g $MgSO_4$	Give IV only	6 hours after last dose or next morning

- $MgSO_4$ 1–2 g, infuse over 1 hour
- $MgSO_4$ 3–6 g, infuse ≤2 g/hour

_____   _____

Physician Signature   Date

Physician order set for the initial management of acute decompensated heart failure in the emergency department/observation unit. AP = anterior/posterior; BNP = b-natriuretic peptide; BUN = blood urea nitrogen; CBC = complete blood cell count; CK = creatine kinase; CK-MB = creatine kinase MB isoenzyme; ECG = electrocardiogram; INR = international normalized ratio; IVP = intravenous push; PT = prothrombin time; PTT = partial thromboplastin time; SBP = systolic blood pressure; SCr = serum creatinine; Clcr = creatinine clearance; ECG = electrocardiogram. Adapted from DiDomenico RJ, Park HY, Southworth MR, et al. Guidelines for acute decompensated heart failure treatment. *Ann Pharmacother.* 2004;38:649–660.

CLINCAL DECISION UNIT ADMISSIONS
ORDERS FOR CONGESTIVE HEART FAILURE

Admit to   ☐ Obtain archival
Primary Dx: Exacerbation of CHF
Secondary Dx:

Condition: _____

VS per CDU Routine Protocol

Nasal Cannula O_2 _____ L/min ☐ Pulse Ox Q _____ hr

☐ Continuous cardiac monitoring

☐ OK to D/C cardiac monitoring during off unit procedures after rule out MI protocol completed.

Optimize Systolic blood pressure: notify MD if too high or low

Optimum Systolic BP = lowest pressure that supports renal function (Urine output >0.5 cc/kg/hr with reasonable BUN/Creatinine) and CNS activity (mentation) without significant or long suffering orthostatic symptoms

Weight done on admission and prior to DC

Strict I & O   ☐ Saline Lock

12 lead EKG and CXR-AP & lateral if not done in ED
Diet: NAS/LAF

Fluid restriction: 1800 cc per 24 hours fluid restriction; Adjust fluid restriction to 1500 cc per 24 hours when Na+ <131 mg/dL

Activity: Up in chair as tolerated/bedside commode; Progress as tolerated to walking in area surrounding Clinical Decision Unit bed space with ECG telemetry monitoring

Insert Foley catheter prn, especially if heavy diuresis interrupts sleep

Patient to view CHF video, and receive *Your Guide to Managing Heart Failure*; RN to complete "Education Assessment" and initiate patient education to meet needs

   ☐ Labs CK-MB, Troponin T q 4 hours × 3;

   ☐ B Natriuretic Peptide Level (BPL) – 2 hours after nesiritide stopped

   ☐ Basic Metabolic Panel and CBC 14 hours after admission or 2 hours before discharge (if planned discharge is before 14 hours)

PRINT NAME _____

MD ATTENDING SIGNATURE_____**BEEPER** _____

Page available in full form on CD   *continued*

☐ Follow potassium nomogram for hypokalemia (see page 159)

☐ Follow magnesium nomogram for hypokalemia (see page 159)

☐ If ejection fraction has never been measured or was measured over 1 year ago and was normal, order echocardiography

☐ Consult: Heart Failure Cardiology Team, if not already done

☐ Nutrition Therapy (if appropriate), may schedule as Out-patient

☐ Social Work (if appropriate for recent/repeat admissions, limited family support; or history of treatment non-compliance)

☐ Initiate intravenous furosemide protocol as follows:

> Give IV Furosemide dose equivalent to prior outpatient *total* daily dose up to 180 mg maximum single dose or → 40 mg IV *if never taken furosemide before*

> Guideline: If normal renal function expect 500 cc urine in 2 hours/onset of action: 5 min.
> If renal insufficiency: expect >250 cc urine in 2 hours

> After 3 hours, if Furosemide is effective but diuresis target has not been reached or if Furosemide has been ineffective in delivering expected 2 hour urine output, double dose of Furosemide and administer IV

> After 6 hours if no diuretic given *and/or* total CDU urine output is <1000 cc, notify MD

> If patient has a very pronounced diuresis response (>2 liters) from diuretics and/or vasodilator therapy, obtain a K+ level

> If resting heart rate <60 or >120 and/or NEW rhythm or conduction disturbances: STAT basic metabolic panel and Mg++ level

> ☐ Ace inhibitor _____ _____ _____
>   DRUG   DOSE   FREQUENCY

> ☐ Nesiritide 2 mcg/kg = _____ mcg bolus if not given in ED, then 0.01 mcg/kg/min = _____ mcg/min

> ☐ BP Monitoring after initiating nesiritide infusion: q15 min 1st hour, then q 4 hours. Notify physician if patient becomes symptomatic or develops a SBP of <85 mmHg.

PRINT NAME _____

MD ATTENDING SIGNATURE _____ **BEEPER** _____

POTASSIUM (Give IV *or* PO dose unless specifically stated)

Level	IV Dose	PO Dose	Recheck K+
3.7–3.9 mEq/dL	20 mEq*	40 mEq*	12 hours or in am
3.4–3.6 mEq/dL	20 mEq × 2 doses*	40 mEq × 2 doses*	6 hours or in am
3.0–3.3 mEq/dL	20 mEq × 4 doses	40 mEq × 3 doses*	4 hours after last dose
Below 3.0 mEq/dL	20 mEq × 6 doses*	Give IV only	1 hr. after last infusion

**Before giving dose, assess last serum Creatinine level. If serum Creatinine level is above 2.5 mg/dL (reflecting renal insufficiency), decrease dose by 50%.

MAGNESIUM (Give IV *or* PO dose unless specifically stated)

Level	IV Dose	PO Dose	Recheck K+
1.9 mg/dL	Give po only	Magnesium Oxide (Uromag) 140 mg	In am
1.3–1.8 mg/dL	*1 g. MgSO$_4$ for every 0.1 mg/dL below 1.9 mg/dL	Give IV only	In am
1.2 mg/dL or below	**8 gms MgSO$_4$	Give IV only	6 hours after last infusion or in am

*Mix 1 to 2 gms MgSO$_4$ in 50 mL of D5W or NaCl 0.9%, infuse over one hour period. Mix 3–6 gms MgSO$_4$ in 150 mL of D5W or NaCl 0.9%; rate should not exceed 2 gms per hour.

**Mix 2 gms MgSO$_4$ in 50 mL of D5W or NaCl 0.9% and infuse over 30 minute period. Repeat 3 more times to achieve adequate level.

If smoker provide smoking cessation education and document educational effort.

PRINT NAME _____

MD ATTENDING SIGNATURE _____**BEEPER** _____

959-1617	Heart Failure OBSERVATION ORDERS - Evidence Based Practice	
TIME	DATE	NOTE: ORDERS MUST BE REVIEWED AND AUTHENTICATED BY RESPONSIBLE PHYSICIAN. Guidelines are not a substitute for the experience and judgment of a physician and are developed to enhance the physician's ability to practice evidence based medicine.

PLACE IN: ☐ Outpatient/Observation status

1. Attending Physician: Consult: Consult: Case Management

2. Diagnosis: Congestive Heart Failure   L.V.E.F. **less than 40%** ☐ Yes ☐ No ☐ Unknown

3. Monitored observation - Vital signs and oxygen saturation every 4 hours and AS NEEDED

4. ☐ Impedence cardiography (ICG) on admission and as needed

5. ☐ Arterial blood gases ☐ Oxygen at   liters per minute per protocol   Other:

6. Old records to floor - include Cardiac Echo report if previously done.

7. Weight on admission and daily

8. Strict Intake and output. Record Intake and Output every   hour(s).   Fluid Restriction: **2 liters every 24 hours**

9. **Labs:** (if not done in E D)

    Comprehensive metabolic panel, Hemogram with platelets and differential, Magnesium, Lipid profile, B-type natriuretic peptide (BNP), urinalysis,

    Digoxin level (if on Digoxin), CPK-MB now, then at 4 hours and 10 hours. Troponin I now and in 10 hours.

10. **Diagnostic Testing**

    Chest X-ray ☐ Portable ☐ PA/ LAT (If not done in ED)   ☐ 2-D Echo to be read by:

    EKG upon arrival, in the morning and as needed for chest pain.

11. **Education:**

    A. Heart Failure education via CHF Education packet

    B. Smoking cessation (for patients who have smoked within 12 months) via CHF Education packet

12. **Diuretics:**

    ☐ Furosemide (Lasix)   milligrams intravenous every   hours ☐ Bumetanide (Bumex)   milligrams intravenous every   hours

13. **Intravenous Vasodilators:**

    ☐ Nesiritide (Natrecor) if systolic blood pressure greater than 90 (use standing orders #959-1488)

14. **Nitrates: Hold for Systolic blood pressure less than:**

    ☐ Nitroglycerin Paste   inches topically every 12 hours   ☐ Isosorbide mononitrate (Imdur)   milligrams by mouth every   hours.

    ☐ Nitroglycerin 0.4mg sublingual AS NEEDED for chest pain or angina

    ☐ Nitroglycerin patch   milligrams per hour apply topical daily, remove at bedtime

15. **ACE Inhibitors:** Contraindication: **Hold for Systolic blood pressure less than:**

    ☐ Captopril (Capoten)   milligrams by mouth every 8 hours   ☐ Lisinopril (Zestril)   milligrams by mouth daily

    ☐ Ramipril (Altace)   milligrams by mouth daily   ☐ Enalapril (Vasotec)   milligrams by mouth every   hour(s)

16. **Angiotensin II Receptor Antagonist:** Contraindication: **Hold for Systolic blood pressure less than:**

    ☐ Valsartan (Diovan)   milligrams by mouth every 12 hours   ☐ Losartan (Cozaar)   milligrams by mouth daily

17. **Beta Blockers:** Contraindication: **Hold for Systolic blood pressure less than:**   **or Heart Rate less than:**

    ☐ Metoprolol (Lopressor)   milligrams by mouth or Intravenous every   hours.

18. ☐ Digoxin (Lanoxin)   milligrams by mouth daily

19. ☐ Aspirin 325 milligrams by mouth daily   ☐ Aspirin 81 milligrams by mouth daily

20. **Electrolyte Replacement**

    ☐ Potassium chloride Protocol (959-1295)   ☐ Magnesium Protocol (959-1494)

21. **Anticoagulation:**

    ☐ Lovenox 30 milligrams subcutaneous twice a day   ☐ Other:

    ☐ Low Dose Heparin Protocol (order # 959-1317AB)

PHYSICIAN SIGNATURE: DATE/TIME:

ALLERGIES: Patient Diagnosis: Height: Weight:

FLORIDA HOSPITAL

EVIDENCE-BASED
PRACTICE
A JOURNEY TO EXCELLENCE

Evidence Based Practice
CHF OBSERVATION ORDERS;
    (7/25/05) R – POD

Page available in full form on CD

BOTSFORD GENERAL HOSPITAL
28050 GRAND RIVER AVENUE
FARMINGTON HILLS, MI 48336-5933

START ——→	DATE:	TIME:

STANDING ORDERS: OBSERVATION HEART FAILURE

1. ☐ ATSO Dr.   ☐ PCU with telemetry

2. ☐ Dr. _____ House Officer beeper #_____ notified
of admission/to see patient upon arrival to floor. Discuss care with Dr. _____
and write further orders.

3. ☐ Consultation: Dr. _____ to consult and participate.

4. ☐ Diagnosis:

5. ☐ Allergies: Weight: _____ Height: _____

6. **Assessment**
   - ☐ Vital signs per protocol
   - ☐ Weight upon admission, in am, and prior to discharge
   - ☐ I & O every shift
   - ☐ O_2 per nasal cannula _____ L/min   ☐ Other
   - ☐ Maintain O_2 saturation > 92%   ☐ AM ambulating pulse ox on RA.
     Notify attending < 92%
   - ☐ Heplock with saline flush every shift

7. **Diet:**
   - ☐ 2 gm Na, low cholesterol   ☐ ADA _____ calories   ☐ Other:
   - ☐ Fluid restriction: ☐ 2 L/day   ☐ 1.5 L/day

8. **Activity:**   ☐ Advance as tolerated

9. **Labs:**
   - ☐ BNP AM
   - ☐ AM lytes, BUN, Creatinine, Mag Phos, TSH, CBC
   - ☐ Lipid profile
     - ☐ fasting   ☐ non-fasting
   - ☐ Dig level
   - ☐ Troponin-I every 4° x 2 after baseline   Time: Baseline: _____
     1. _____
     2. _____
   - ☐ Daily PT/INR (if on Coumadin)

10. **Tests:**
    - ☐ AM ECG r/o ischemia
    - ☐ 2D mode echo with colorflow doppler
    - ☐ AM CXR r/o CHF

Physician Signature:

Beeper #:

USE ONLY BALLPOINT PEN

MATCH

PATIENT

IDENTITY

8/3/05

Page available in full form on CD

11. **Medications:**
- [ ] Zestril _____ mg po every day   hold if SBP < 90 mmHg
- [ ] Hydralazine: _____   hold if SBP < 100 mmHg
- [ ] Lopressor _____ mg po BID   hold if AR < 60 BPM
  - [ ] Coreg: _____ mg po BID
  - [ ] Toprol XL _____ mg po every day
- [ ] Lasix: _____ mg IV every _____
- [ ] Bumex _____ mg IV every _____
- [ ] ASA 325mg every day
- [ ] ASA 162mg every day
- [ ] ASA 81mg every day
- [ ] Zocor _____ mg po every HS
- [ ] Imdur _____ mg po every day
- [ ] IV: 25mg Nitroglycerin in 250cc D$_5$W at 10 mcg/min. Titrate every 2 hours
  - Double the dose to Maintain Systolic BP > 100

Anticoagulation Therapy:
- [ ] Daily Coumadin:
- [ ] Lovenox 1 mg/kg subcutaneous every 12 hours
- [ ] Heparin 5,000 units subcutaneous b.i.d. x _____ doses
- [ ] IV: 25,000 units Heparin in 250cc D$_5$W at 10cc/hour
  - Bolus: Heparin _____ units IVP prior to starting drip

    Adjust per Nomogram

	APTT (seconds)	Bolus Dose (Units)	Stop Infusion (Minutes)	Rate Change (cc/hour)	Repeat APTT
	< 40	3,000	0 min.	+ 1 cc/hour	6 hours
	40 - 49	0	0 min.	+ 1 cc/hour	6 hours
Target →	50 - 75	0	0 min.	0 (no change)	next AM
	76 - 85	0	0 min.	- 1 cc/hour	next AM
	86 - 100	0	30 min.	- 1 cc/hour	6 hours
	100 - 120	0	60 min.	- 2 cc/hour	6 hours
	> 120	0	60 min.	- 3 cc/hour	6 hours

- [ ] Other medication:

12. [ ] **Miscellaneous:**
- [ ] Stress test
  - [ ] Dob stress echo
  - [ ] Stress Echo
  - [ ] Persantine cardiolite
- [ ] NPO after midnight
- [ ] Continuing Care to evaluate home care needs
- [ ] Provide Heart Failure Patient booklet to patient
- [ ] Old chart to floor

MATCH

PATIENT

IDENTITY

Physician Signature:

Beeper #:

USE ONLY BALLPOINT PEN

8/3/05

Page available in full form on CD

CHF Rapid Diagnosis and Treatment Center Orders

1. **Admit to Rapid Diagnosis and Treatment Center (RDTC)** (for 12 hour time period, then reassess: maximum 23 hours)
2. **Diagnosis:** Decompensated Heart Failure
3. *Notify appropriate nurse at time of patient's admission to RDTC* (based on attached schedule)
4. **Consult:** Social Services
5. **Nursing Care:**
   1. Vital Signs Q 1 hour × 4, then Q 2 hours.
   2. Continuous cardiac monitor
   3. Weight upon admission: _____ kg
   4. Record cardiac rhythm and I&Os with vital signs (Q1 hour × 4, then Q2 hrs)
   5. Foley catheter to gravity drain (at nurse's discretion/patient's decision)
   6. IV: Heplock
   7. Show Heart Failure video (located at Nurse's Station)
6. **Activity:**
   ☐ Bedrest
   ☐ Bathroom privileges
7. **Nutrition:**
   1. 2 g Na restricted cardiac diet
   2. Oral fluid restriction of 500 cc over 14 hours
8. **Respiratory Care:**
   1. O_2 per nasal canula @ _____ L/min.
   2. Continuous pulse oximetry
   3. May wean oxygen to maintain pulse ox >93%
   4. Record FIO_2 and pulse ox with VS (Q 1 hr × 4, then Q 2 hrs)
9. **Notify MD for:**
   – Chest pain
   – T >101°F PO
   – SBP >180 mmHg or <90 mmHg
   – DBP >110 mmHg or <50 mmHg
   – HR >120 bpm or <60 bpm, or change in rhythm
   – RR >25 or <10
   – Pulse ox <90% or any increase in oxygen requirement
   – Urine output <500 ml after 2 hours

10. **Tests:**
    1. Laboratory:
       a. CBC
       b. EP1
          Baseline Electrolyte panel (date and time due) _____
          6 hour Electrolyte panel (date and time due)_____
          12 hour Electrolyte panel (date and time due)_____
          Disposition/discharge EP1 (date and time due)_____
       c. Baseline CK, CK-MB, Troponin (if not already sent in ED)
          3 hour CK, CK-MB, Troponin (date and time due)_____
          6 hour CK, CK-MB, Troponin (date and time due)_____
       d. Baseline BNP (if not already sent in ED)
          6–12 hour BNP level (date and time due)_____
          Disposition BNP level (date and time due)_____
       e. Digoxin level (if patient on Digoxin and not already sent in ED)
    2. Diagnostic: (*Notify MD when complete*)
       a. Echocardiogram for "Shortness of Breath" (if not done in last 6 months)
          Call to schedule
       b. Rest SPECT scan (if RDTC attending deems necessary) × 1
          Call to schedule
11. **Medications Upon Arrival to RDTC**
    1. Pneumovax 0.5 ml × 1 per ED standards
    2. Hold all Beta blockers
    3. Apply Nitroglycerin 2% ointment topical _____ inch(es) Q 6 hours
    4. Aspirin 325 mg PO/NG/PR × 1 (if not given in ED)
    5. ACE Inhibitor (ACEI)
       a) If patient currently takes an ACEI at home, administer patient's home ACEI:_____ _____ mg × 1 (If their home ACEI is not on formulary, call pharmacy to find out the Captopril equivalent, give only if creatinine <1.8
          Along with oral ACEI, may also give:
          ☐ Enalaprilat 1.25 mg IV ×1
          OR
       b) If not currently taking an ACEI at home, choose ONE from below:
          ☐ Captopril 12.5 mg PO tid (if pt. is ACEI naïve/noncompliant)
          OR
          ☐ Losartan 25 mg PO × 1 (if intolerant to ACEI)

    6. Metolazone (only if patient currently takes this at home)
       a) ☐ 2.5 mg PO × 1
          OR
       b) ☐ 5 mg PO × 1
    7. **Furosemide *OR* Torsemide regimen**
       – Give whichever medication they are taking at home
       – If not on a loop diuretic, give Furosemide

Page available in full form on CD

a) **Furosemide**
- *If not already given in the ED*
- *Up to 2× daily home dose*
- *Or 40 mg IV if not on Furosemide at home*

(*MD check dose ordered*)
☐ Furosemide 40 mg IVP × 1
☐ Furosemide 80 mg IVP × 1
☐ Furosemide 120 mg IVPB over 30–60 minutes × 1
☐ Furosemide 160 mg IVPB over 30–60 minutes × 1

OR

b) **Torsemide**
- *Only if taking this at home, same as home dose*
- *If patient unable to tolerate PO contact pharmacy to have them convert Torsemide dose to Furosemide IV dose*

(*MD check dose ordered*)
☐ Torsemide 20 mg PO × 1
☐ Torsemide 40 mg PO × 1
☐ Torsemide 80 mg PO × 1
☐ Torsemide 100 mg PO × 1

8. Home Medications to be given in RDTC: (list)
☐ _____
☐ _____
☐ _____
☐ _____
☐ _____
☐ _____
☐ _____

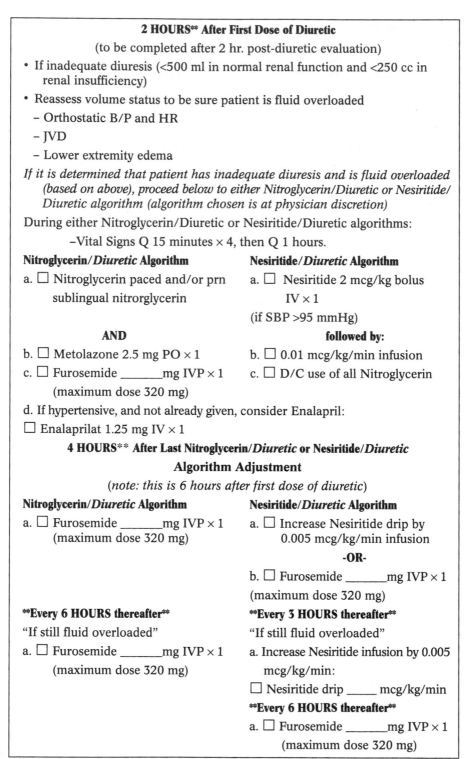

2 HOURS After First Dose of Diuretic**

(to be completed after 2 hr. post-diuretic evaluation)

- If inadequate diuresis (<500 ml in normal renal function and <250 cc in renal insufficiency)
- Reassess volume status to be sure patient is fluid overloaded
  - Orthostatic B/P and HR
  - JVD
  - Lower extremity edema

If it is determined that patient has inadequate diuresis and is fluid overloaded (based on above), proceed below to either Nitroglycerin/Diuretic or Nesiritide/ Diuretic algorithm (algorithm chosen is at physician discretion)

During either Nitroglycerin/Diuretic or Nesiritide/Diuretic algorithms:

–Vital Signs Q 15 minutes × 4, then Q 1 hours.

Nitroglycerin/*Diuretic* Algorithm

a. ☐ Nitroglycerin paced and/or prn sublingual nitrorglycerin

AND

b. ☐ Metolazone 2.5 mg PO × 1
c. ☐ Furosemide _____ mg IVP × 1
(maximum dose 320 mg)

Nesiritide/*Diuretic* Algorithm

a. ☐ Nesiritide 2 mcg/kg bolus
  IV × 1
(if SBP >95 mmHg)

followed by:

b. ☐ 0.01 mcg/kg/min infusion
c. ☐ D/C use of all Nitroglycerin

d. If hypertensive, and not already given, consider Enalapril:
☐ Enalaprilat 1.25 mg IV × 1

4 HOURS After Last Nitroglycerin/*Diuretic* or Nesiritide/*Diuretic***

Algorithm Adjustment

(note: this is 6 hours after first dose of diuretic)

Nitroglycerin/*Diuretic* Algorithm

a. ☐ Furosemide _____ mg IVP × 1
(maximum dose 320 mg)

Nesiritide/*Diuretic* Algorithm

a. ☐ Increase Nesiritide drip by 0.005 mcg/kg/min infusion

-OR-

b. ☐ Furosemide _____ mg IVP × 1
(maximum dose 320 mg)

Every 6 HOURS thereafter

"If still fluid overloaded"

a. ☐ Furosemide _____ mg IVP × 1
(maximum dose 320 mg)

Every 3 HOURS thereafter

"If still fluid overloaded"

a. Increase Nesiritide infusion by 0.005 mcg/kg/min:

☐ Nesiritide drip _____ mcg/kg/min

Every 6 HOURS thereafter

a. ☐ Furosemide _____ mg IVP × 1
(maximum dose 320 mg)

Page available in full form on CD

12. **PRN Medications**
    1. Morphine 2–5 mg IVP Q3 hours prn per MD's discretion
    2. Albuterol 0.5 cc in 3 cc NS nebulized Q1 hour PRN wheezing
    3. Acetaminophen 650 mg PO/PR Q4 hours PRN fever >101
    4. Potassium Replacement Sliding Scale
       - Potassium (Reference Range 3.5–5 mg/dl)
       - Peripheral line: Infuse at 10 mEq/hr
       - Recheck K+ level 1 hour after administration of replacements
       - DO NOT give more than 60 mEq KCL w/o rechecking K+ level

Serum Potassium Level (mg/dl)	IV Potassium Chloride Dose**
3.7–4.0	20 mEq KCL PO (*preferred*) or IVPB
3.4–3.6	40 mEq KCL PO (*preferred*) or IVPB
3.0–3.3	60 mEq KCL PO (*preferred*) or IVPB
<3.0	notify MD

    5. Magnesium Replacement Sliding Scale
       - Magnesium (Reference Range 1.3–2.1 mg/dl)
         a. If Magnesium level <1.6 then Magnesium Sulfate 5 g IVPB (infuse over five hours)
13. **Orders Prior to Discharge**
    1. Discharge weight
    2. Discharge vital signs

CHF Rapid Diagnosis and Treatment Center Orders

1. **Contact Cardiology fellow/attending to discuss discharge**
2. **Follow up in Heart Failure Clinic:** (Heart Failure Clinic Phone number: xxx-xxxx)

    Date _____ Time _____

3. **Pneumovax Received** ☐ **No**   ☐ **Yes** **Date/time** _____
4. **Discharge Medications**

    ☐ ACEI _____

    ☐ Diuretic _____

    ☐ Beta-Blocker_____
    (1/2 original dose patient was taking at home: only if recommended by Cardiologist)

    ☐ ARB _____

    ☐ Digoxin _____

    ☐ KCl _____

    ☐ Spironolactone _____

    ☐ Non-cardiac home _____
    medications

    _____

    _____

    ☐ Other _____

    _____

5. **Patients should return to the Emergency Department for:**
    a. Worsening breathing
    b. Chest pain
    c. Weight gain
    d. Worsening leg swelling

Other Instructions: _____

_____

_____

_____

_____

_____

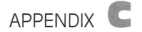
PATIENT DISCHARGE INSTRUCTIONS

Heart Failure Patient Information

What Is Heart Failure?

Heart failure is the inability of the heart muscle to pump effectively. In heart failure, the heart is unable to supply enough blood to allow normal body function. When the heart muscle doesn't squeeze strongly enough, blood can back up into the heart and lungs. Increased pressure then forces fluid from the blood into the breathing spaces of the lungs as well as into other places. This congestion of tissues with fluid is what gives the condition its name. When you have heart failure, it does not mean that your heart has stopped pumping or beating or has completely failed.

Currently, your symptoms may seriously limit your activities. You may feel frightened by your diagnosis. You also may feel discouraged about your treatment plan. But there are outstanding treatments for heart failure that can help you feel better, stay out of the hospital, and live longer. You can take control of heart failure by understanding and carefully following your treatment plan.

What Are the Signs and Symptoms?

As a heart failure patient, you may experience some or all of the following:
- Shortness of breath
- Fatigue, tiredness, loss of energy
- Loss of appetite, abdominal discomfort
- Abdominal bloating (stomach swelling)
- Swollen ankles or legs
- Weight gain (two to three pounds over a few days)

What Should I Do If My Symptoms Worsen?

If you ever have questions about your symptoms or medications, call your doctor. In an emergency, call 911 and ask the paramedics to take you to the nearest emergency room. Call your physician if you experience any of the following:
- Chest pain/pressure that is new or present at rest, or if there is a change in the pattern of the pain. If you experience chest pain, take sublingual nitroglycerin (under your tongue) as prescribed, one pill every five minutes for up to three pills, and lie down. If pain is still unrelieved, call 911 or go to the nearest emergency room, and notify your physician.
- Difficulty breathing, shortness of breath at rest
- Dizziness, feeling faint, or passing out
- Swelling of the feet, ankles, or lower legs
- Palpitations, fast or irregular heartbeats
- Weight gain of greater than two pounds overnight or three to four pounds in a week
- Nausea or vomiting
- Severe leg cramping (may be due to a low potassium level in the body)
- Decrease in exercise tolerance

If you ever have any questions about your medications, call your doctor or nurse. Do not stop taking any medications on your own without advising your doctor.

What Else Can I Do?

Daily Weighings

It is recommended that you monitor your daily weight. Daily weighings are the best way to determine if you are retaining fluid. If your heart isn't pumping properly, fluid may begin to accumulate in your body, and this results in an increase in weight. If you eat too much salt or drink too much fluid, your weight can increase. It is very important that you weigh yourself each day and record your weight on a weight chart. Daily weighings should be done at the same time every day (for example, in the morning after you urinate, before you eat breakfast), wearing the same amount of clothing, and then recorded on your weight chart. Gaining two pounds overnight or three to four pounds in a week is abnormal and may be the earliest sign of fluid retention. If this occurs, you should follow the instructions to increase your diuretic (water pill) dose, or call your physician/nurse and they will make adjustments in your diuretic dose and possibly your potassium dose.

Know and Take Your Medications

Your heart failure will be treated with a combination of medications, changes in your salt and fluid intake, and close monitoring. These medications can help to strengthen your heart muscle and prevent it from dilating (enlarging) further. They can help make you feel better, do more activities, decrease the likelihood you will require hospitalization, and may help you to live longer.

Because you will be treated with a number of different medications, it is very important that you know your medications well. Your medications are likely to have changed while you were in the hospital, with new ones added, old ones stopped, and the doses adjusted. It is essential that you understand your new medication regimen exactly prior to hospital discharge.

It is important that you keep an updated list of all the medications you take and keep this list with you at all times. If you are not sure of the medications and doses you are taking, it is difficult for the doctor to make adjustments when needed. Use of a pill organizer may be helpful in planning which medicines need to be taken each day so that doses are not missed. Additionally, you should be familiar with what your pills look like in size and color.

Three classes of medications have been shown to allow heart failure patients to live longer:
- ACE inhibitors
- Beta-blockers
- Aldosterone antagonists

A standard regimen often includes an ACE inhibitor, a Beta-blocker, spironolactone, and a loop diuretic. Medications are used to improve the heart function, decrease salt and water retention, reduce symptoms, improve exercise tolerance, and improve rates of survival. These medications are very important to adequately treat this condition. It is essential that you take them as prescribed and not let your prescriptions run out. Also, if you are taking a trip, be sure you have an adequate supply of medications.

If you have any new symptoms or side effects with a medication, discuss them with your physician. If you ever have any questions about your medications, call your doctor or nurse. Do not stop taking any medications on your own without advising your doctor.

Page available in full form on CD

How Does My Diet Have to Change?

It is recommended you follow a two-gram sodium diet. Heart failure patients should take in no more than 2000 milligrams (mgs) of sodium a day. Salt is about 40 percent sodium and is among the top sources of sodium in the average diet. Sodium will cause fluid to be retained in your body, resulting in worsening heart failure. Even a pinch of salt added to foods can make it hard to stay within your daily sodium restriction. You should find it easy to adjust to a low-sodium diet if you follow these guidelines:

- Do not add salt to your food at the table. Instead, season with fresh or dried herbs, garlic, onion, or lemon. Avoid condiments with salt in their names. Garlic powder and onion powder do not contain salt.
- Buy fresh fruits and vegetables. These do not have added salt.
- Avoid convenience foods (e.g., canned, frozen, or deli food). These frequently have added salt.
- Check labels for words that indicate added sodium (e.g., salt, sodium, monosodium glutamate [MSG], sodium chloride [NaCl]). Such products should be avoided as they are all forms of sodium. Be cautious about low-salt/low-sodium products because even products labeled light or $\frac{1}{3}$ less may be high in sodium.
- When eating out, ask that foods be prepared without salt or salty seasonings such as teriyaki sauce, soy sauce, salad dressings, BBQ sauce, and monosodium glutamate. You should also order the sauces on the side so you can control how much you use.
- You may use a salt substitute. But do not use large quantities of this product because salt substitutes have a high potassium content and may alter your blood potassium level.
- Check with your physician before taking other medications that may contain large amounts of sodium (e.g., Alka-Seltzer®, antacids, laxatives).

In addition to a low-salt diet, your doctor also may recommend that you be on a low-fat, low-cholesterol, or anti-diabetic diet. Please ask your doctor, nurse, or dietician for other instructions about low-sodium and low-fat diets.

Fluid Restriction

This is done to reduce fluid retention. Your doctor may request that you restrict your daily fluid intake to two quarts (slightly less than two liters) a day, or perhaps even less if you have been having more problems with fluid retention. This is equivalent to eight eight-ounce glasses a day. It is important to measure all liquids taken in over a 24-hour period, including soups, ice cream, yogurt, popsicles, and gelatins. Some fruits (e.g., melons and citrus fruits) have a high water content and should not be consumed in large quantities. If you eat large amounts of fruit, you need to count this as part of your fluid intake and adjust the amount of fluid you drink.

Alcohol

Alcohol and heart failure are a bad combination. Alcohol damages cardiac cells and can lead to a further deterioration and weakness of the heart muscle. Even as much as a glass of wine or one drink a few times a week can be detrimental to your heart. As a general rule, you should not consume any alcoholic beverages.

Cigarette Smoking

You are advised to stop smoking completely.

Research indicates that smoking increases the risk of premature heart disease three- to sixfold and causes lung damage. Smoking reduces the amount of oxygen in your blood, increases your heart rate, constricts your blood vessels, and increases your blood pressure. Smoking can worsen heart

failure, so it is strongly recommended that you not smoke. Smoking cessation
programs and nicotine-replacement therapy can help you quit. If you are interested in further
information about quitting, ask your physician.

What Should My Activity Level Be?

Discuss with your physician whether an exercise program is right for you. In many cases, it will be
recommended that you begin an exercise program.

Exercise may be beneficial for patients with heart failure. Studies still are evaluating whether this
helps heart failure patients live longer. Exercise may make you feel better, allow you to accomplish
more, and make routine daily activities easier to do. While aerobic exercise may be recommended,
in general, patients with more advanced heart failure should avoid resistance training and lifting
more than 10 lbs.

How Do I Start an Exercise Program?

- Discuss with your physician before starting to exercise.
- Start slowly. It will take time for your heart, muscles, tendons, and bones to build strength.
- Start by walking for five minutes a day, six to seven days a week. Gradually increase your
  activity level each week. When five minutes of exercise becomes easy, increase to ten minutes
  daily. When ten minutes becomes easy, increase to 15 minutes daily, etc.
- When you get to 30 minutes a day of exercise, you should try to increase the pace by covering
  a greater distance in the 30-minute time period.
- Develop a weekly exercise schedule that works with your daily schedule.
- If you miss exercising for a couple of days, you may have to exercise at a lower level for a
  few days and progressively work back up to your former level.
- Once you are walking 30 minutes a day, you can switch to other aerobic activities such as
  biking or swimming.

What About Sex?

Sexual activity, like most physical activity, means added work for your heart. Studies have shown
that sexual intercourse requires about the same amount of energy as climbing one to two flights of
stairs or walking briskly. The guidelines for sexual activity are the same as for any other exercise —
as tolerated. Sexual activity should occur in a relaxed environment to reduce the stress on your
heart. Try to avoid positions where you support your weight with your arms for prolonged periods.
If you are having any sexual difficulties and/or performance problems, please do not hesitate to
discuss these with your physician or nurse.

What Is My Follow-Up?

It is recommended that you have a follow-up appointment with your doctor within 14 days of being
discharged from the hospital with heart failure.

You should make sure that you have appointments scheduled with your doctors before you leave the
hospital. Don't miss your appointments, or if you do, make sure to reschedule. Continuation of the
medications to treat your heart failure can markedly improve how well you do. It is important that you
follow up with your doctor and continue the use of the beneficial therapies that were started while
you were in the hospital. One of the major reasons patients are readmitted to the hospital is that they
did not continue to take their heart medications or did not follow a low-salt diet.

- Follow your doctor's advice.
- Take your medications as advised.

- Eat a low, two gram sodium diet, restrict your fluid intake, keep a healthy body weight.
- Keep your doctor appointments.
- Monitor your weight, keep a record of your daily weighings.
- If you smoke, stop. Complete cessation of smoking is advised.

Understanding Your Medications

ACE Inhibitors
My ACE inhibitor is: _____

ACE inhibitors work by blocking some of the harmful substances that the body produces. As a result, they help to relax blood vessels (vasodilator), reduce blood pressure, and make it easier for the heart to work. Over the long term, ACE inhibitors may improve symptoms and exercise tolerance, help to stabilize the heart and kidneys, prevent hospitalizations, improve quality of life, and increase lifespan.

TIP   One of the most common side effects of these drugs includes lightheadedness. This is usually due to a reduction in blood pressure. Should this occur and you are on a long-acting ACE inhibitor that is taken only once daily, be sure to take the drug just prior to bedtime. This will help to reduce the lightheadedness. Overall, these drugs are very well tolerated.

TIP   In a few patients, these drugs can cause a dry cough. If this occurs, your doctor may substitute the ACE inhibitor for a similar type of drug that will not cause a cough; these are called angiotensin receptor blockers (ARBs).

TIP   Because these drugs may affect the kidneys and raise blood potassium levels, routine blood tests should be taken to monitor your kidney function and blood potassium levels.

Beta-blockers
My beta-blocker is:_____

Beta-blockers block hormones that are harmful to the heart. They act by slowing the heart rate and reducing the workload on the heart. They also reduce blood pressure. Beta-blockers may reduce the progression of heart disease, help to improve the pumping function of the heart, reduce hospitalizations, improve quality of life, and increase lifespan.

TIP   Beta-blockers are very effective drugs but can be a little tricky to use. They are started at a low dose when you are in a relatively stable state. The dose will be increased slowly over time.

TIP   Side effects of these drugs sometimes can occur and include fatigue, lightheadedness, sexual problems such as erectile dysfunction, and on occasion, shortness of breath and fluid retention. These side effects often resolve on their own or with adjustments in the dose of beta-blocker or your other medicines. Should you experience any side effects, it is important to speak with your doctor or nurse and try to "work through" these symptoms (do not stop taking the medicines unless advised to by a healthcare professional). Overall, these drugs are very well tolerated.

Page available in full form on CD

Aldosterone Antagonists

My aldosterone antagonist is: _____

Aldosterone antagonists work by helping the kidneys get rid of sodium and water and by blocking some of the body's own harmful hormones. In addition to helping to prevent fluid retention, the drug improves symptoms, reduces hospitalizations, and increases lifespan in patients who have at least a moderate degree of heart failure.

TIP   Aldosterone antagonists may cause the potassium level in the blood to increase and can occasionally "dry" the kidneys a bit. As such, routine blood tests should be monitored while you are on these drugs. Depending on your potassium level, you may be asked to avoid foods that have a lot of potassium in them (see "Diuretics"). Other sources of potassium include salt substitutes and some vitamins.

TIP   Side effects of spironolactone can include breast enlargement or tenderness, even in men. If either occurs and is bothersome, an adjustment in the dose may be necessary to eliminate these effects.

Diuretics (water pills)

My diuretic(s) is(are): _____

Diuretics help to eliminate the buildup of water and sodium in areas of the body such as the lungs, liver, stomach, and legs. By doing so, they can make it easier for the heart to pump and reduce any difficulty in breathing that you may experience if fluid builds up. You may be on more than one diuretic.

TIP   As you will likely experience an increase in urine output after taking these drugs, be sure to take them at the most convenient times — e.g., when you will be at home or have easy bathroom access. Although it is OK to adjust the time of day that you take diuretics, you should never just "skip" taking them for convenience.

TIP   Some diuretics cause the body to lose potassium. One of the symptoms of low potassium includes muscle cramps. You may be asked to eat more potassium-rich foods (bananas, oranges, and other fruits and vegetables), or you may require a potassium pill while on certain diuretics.

TIP   Should you experience another illness that also deprives your body of fluid (nausea, vomiting, diarrhea, fever, or reduced food intake), let your doctor or nurse know, as you may be more prone to getting dehydrated (dry) while on diuretics. Symptoms of dehydration include dizziness, weakness, and increase in thirst.

Digitalis (Digoxin®, Lanoxin®, Digitek®)

Digitalis helps the heart pump more strongly and may also help control irregular heart rhythms. This may result in an improvement in symptoms.

TIP   Digitalis works effectively but can have side effects if you have too much in your blood. On occasion, a blood test may be required to measure the level of the drug. Symptoms to notify your doctor or nurse of include nausea, vomiting or diarrhea, stomach pain or reduced appetite, slow heart rate, confusion, dizziness, or blurred vision (including yellow, green, or white "halos").

Adhere®

Page available in full form on CD

OBSERVATION UNIT DISCHARGE GUIDELINES

Treating heart failure (HF) in the observation unit represents an opportunity for short (<24 hours) intensive therapy in patients who are unlikely to require prolonged hospitalization. In parallel with treatment, monitoring and diagnostic strategies are needed to aid the assessment of potential precipitants of the patient's current presentation. Once diagnostic and therapeutic goals have been attained, discharge can be considered. A significant percentage of patients will not meet targeted goals within the time frame available for observation unit therapy. In this population, inpatient admission for continued therapy will be necessary. Successful discharge may require some or all of the following:

- Patient reports subjective improvement
- Ambulatory, without long suffering orthostasis
- Resting HR <100 beats/min, BP >80 mmHg
- Total urine output >1 L, and >30 cc/hr or 0.5 cc/kg/hr
- Room air O_2 sat >90% (unless on home O_2)
- No CKMB >8.8 ng/ml, or troponin T >0.1
- No ischemic CP or clinically significant arrhythmia
- Stable electrolyte profile

REFERENCES

Peacock WF 4th, Remer EE, Aponte J, Moffa DA, Emerman CE, Albert NM. Effective observation unit treatment of decompensated heart failure. *Congest Heart Fail.* 2002 Mar–Apr;8:68–73.

EMERGENCY DEPARTMENT DISCHARGE GUIDELINES

Emergency department (ED) disposition may be considered from the perspective of an estimate of the acuity of the patient's initial hemodynamic and symptomatic presentation. It is suggested that certain clinical features should then alter the initial acuity estimate. The following are reasonable factors to consider in the disposition decision, although many of the parameters have not been extensively studied. When possible, the supporting literature is referenced.

It should be noted that in the current state of the art, a "low-risk" patient has not been identified, and the absence of high-risk features to develop a low-risk profile is only an extrapolation. In addition, every recommendation must be interpreted with the patient's baseline status in mind. Not every patient will meet all of these criteria.

Appropriate discharge from the ED must be combined with adequate follow-up. Instruction on diet recommendations, medication schedules, and the importance of tracking body weight are important in preventing readmission.

High-risk features

1. New-onset heart failure (HF)[1]
2. Ischemic changes or positive cardiac markers on electrocardiogram (ECG)[2,3]
3. Low serum sodium[4,5]
4. Increased respiratiory rate[6]
5. Low systolic blood pressure (SBP)[7-9]
6. Age >70[1]
7. Chest pain[1]
8. Elevated creatinine[8,10]
9. Poor diuresis at 4 hours[3]
10. Pulmonary edema on chest x-ray[10]
11. Severe comorbidities[4]
12. Electrolyte abnormalities
13. Syncope[11]
14. Valvular disease[1]
15. Hemoglobin <10[12]

Low-risk features (ie, consider discharge if)

1. Lack of high-risk features
2. Normal vital signs and symptomatic improvement after treatment
3. Good social support and outpatient follow-up
4. Normal laboratory parameters (electrolytes, cardiac markers)

Criteria	Rationale and References

Presenting Complaint

No chest pain that would raise concern for acute coronary syndrome (ACS)[13]	Patients with HF have multiple risk factors for ACS. The presence of chest pain, raising concern for ACS, mandates serial cardiac injury marker testing. ACS has been reported to be the trigger for up to 25% of all HF readmissions.
History not suspicious for deep vein thrombosis (DVT) or pulmonary embolism[14]	Patients with HF are at increased risk for DVT and subsequent DVT. In patients where the exact cause of dyspnea is uncertain, especially if the B-type natriuretic peptide (BNP) level is not conclusive, admission is necessary.
No evidence of infection[13]	Patients with a history of HF who have concomitant infection are at increased risk for decompensation. One study reported that respiratory infection was the trigger for HF readmission in 10% of all cases.

Quality-of-Life Indicators

Improvement in dyspnea[15]	The assessment of dyspnea has been shown to correlate with hemodynamic status in clinical trials. Although subjective, the measurement of dyspnea on a 7-point scale or a 3-point scale is a validated outcome measure. No study has evaluated this as an endpoint in an observation unit.
Ability to ambulate without dyspnea above baseline[16]	Although there is no trial that has assessed this measure in an observation unit setting, it effectively is an inexpensive 6-minute exercise test. The distance that a patient can ambulate in a 6 minute period without excessive dyspnea and fatigue has been shown to correlate with long-term mortality. Many comorbid illnesses can affect this outcome measure, hence it is important to assess a change from baseline.

Hemodynamic/Clinical Parameters

SBP <160 mm Hg, >90 mm Hg[17]	Although in the initial presentation of patients with decompensated HF a hypertensive response is adaptive, persistent elevation of SBP can correlate with increased risk of worsening renal function. This deterioration of renal function clearly correlates with morbidity and mortality. Adjustment of medications to prevent hypertension is essential prior to discharge. The cut-off of SBP >160 is not ideal; however, it is the value that has been studied.

Page available in full form on CD

Criteria	Rationale and References
	Patients should be able ambulate without dizziness if their SBP is around 90 mmHg.
No S₃ on auscultation[18]	Of all the clinical examination findings, the presence of an S_3 is most suggestive of acute decompensation.
Improvement in thoracic electrical bioimpedance measurements[19]	Multiple studies have shown that bioimpedance measurements can aid in the diagnosis of HF. Because these measurements correlate with a patient's hemodynamic parameters, it may be a useful measurement in the early management of HF patients. In addition, bioimpedance is utilized in the outpatient setting, so the patient's baseline values may be known. Currently there are no studies that track changes in bioimpedance values in ED patients and assess the impact on patient outcomes.
Oxygen saturation >90%	No data exist to support this value; however, it is reasonable to only discharge patients who are able to maintain their oxygen saturations. Transient night-time drops in oxygen saturations are common because HF is associated with an increased prevalence of obstructive sleep apnea. Therefore, pulse oximetry as a discharge criterion should be assessed when the patient is awake.
Urine output >1 L	Although there are no studies that compare the amount of urine output with outcomes, intuitively this makes sense. Clinically, 1 L appears to be a significant amount.
Decrease in weight/ return to dry weight	Dry weight is often one of the only baseline parameters that we know in the ED. Return to the patient's dry weight can slow the progression of the disease process; however, "over-shooting" this parameter can lead to hypotension and hypoperfusion of vital organs.
No ischemic changes on ECG and no arrhythmias[20]	The most common cause of death in HF patients is ventricular arrhythmia. In patients with HF, the presence of a prolonged QRS >120 msec, left ventricular hypertrophy, and left bundle branch block are predictors of poor outcome. However, there are no data to support that any of these findings affect short-term outcome.
	The presence of new ischemic changes is indicative of ACS and mandates admission to the hospital. Atrial fibrillation is a common trigger of HF decompensation.

Page available in full form on CD

Criteria	Rationale and References
Laboratory Measurements	
BNP levels[21]	Patients with levels greater than 20% of their baseline may have an acute decompensation. Although there is no study that identifies an exact percentage above baseline, this value accounts for any variation in renal function or assay imprecision.
	Studies have shown that a decline in BNP levels is associated with improved morbidity and decreased hospital readmission rate. No study has looked at the change in BNP levels in the <23 hours timeframe.
Stable creatinine[17]	Recent study has shown that an increase in creatinine level of >0.3 mg/dl from hospital admission correlates with in-hospital death, complications, and length of stay. The presence of worsening renal insufficiency as defined by a creatinine change >0.3 mg/dl from prior values is concerning and in patients with acute decompensation may be considered a marker of the need for admission.
Stable or declining troponin level[22]	Elevated troponin levels have been shown to be predictive of long-term prognosis in HF patients. Patients with severe HF may have chronically elevated levels. However, a rise in troponin levels during an observation unit stay should provoke concern and may reflect inadequacy of treatment or the presence of ACS.
Return to normal or baseline of electrolytes and blood urea nitrogen (BUN)[23]	A sodium level of <136 mEq/L has been shown to correlate with 30-day and 1-year mortality. In addition, an elevated BUN has also been shown to correlate with 30-day and 1-year mortality. Some studies have reported that an increased risk of morbidity is associated with a BUN >50 mg/dl.
	In patients with normal serum sodium levels and BUN levels at baseline, a decrease in sodium <136 mEq/L should be an indicator of the need for admission.

REFERENCES

1. Esdaile JM, Horwitz RI, Levinton C, et al. Response to initial therapy and new onset as predictors of prognosis in patients hospitalized with congestive heart failure. *Clin Invest Med*. 1992;15:122–131.

2. Selker HP, Griffith JL, D'Agostino RB. A time-insensitive predictive instrument for acute hospital mortality due to congestive heart failure: development, testing, and use for comparing hospitals: a multicenter study. *Med Care*. 1994;32:1040–1052.

3. Katz MH, Nicholson BW, Singer DE, et al. The triage decision in pulmonary edema. *J Gen Intern Med*. 1988;3:533–539.

4. Chin MH, Goldman L. Correlates of major complications or death in patients admitted to the hospital with congestive heart failure. *Arch Intern Med*. 1996;156:1814–1820.

5. Villacorta H, Rocha N, Cardoso R, et al. [Hospital outcome and short-term follow-up of elderly patients presenting to the emergency unit with congestive heart failure.] *Arq Bras Cardiol*. 1998;70:167–171. Portuguese.

6. Rame JE, Sheffield MA, Dries OL, et al. Outcomes after emergency department discharge with a primary diagnosis of heart failure. *Am Heart J*. 2001;142:714–719.

7. Chin MH, Goldman L. Correlates of early hospital readmission or death in patients with congestive heart failure. *Am J Cardiol*. 1997;79:1640–1644.

8. Cowie MR, Wood DA, Coats AJ, et al. Survival of patients with a new diagnosis of heart failure: a population based study. *Heart*. 2000;83:505–510.

9. Plotnick GD, Kelemen MH, Garrett RB, et al. Acute cardiogenic pulmonary edema in the elderly: factors predicting in-hospital and one-year mortality. *South Med J*. 1982;75:565–569.

10. Butler J, Hanumanthu S, Chomsky D, Wilson JR. Frequency of low-risk hospital admissions for heart failure. *Am J Cardiol*. 1998;81:41–44.

11. Konstam M, Dracup K, Baker D. Heart failure: evaluation and care of patients with left ventricular systolic dysfunction. *J Cardiac Fail*. 1995;1:183–187.

12. Fonarow GC, Adams KF, Abraham WT, for the ADHERE Investigators. Risk Stratification for In-Hospital Mortality in Heart Failure Using Classification and Regression Tree (CART) Methodology: Analysis of 33,046 Patients in the ADHERE Registry. *JCF*. 2003;9:S79.

13. Khand AU, Gemmell I, Rankin AC, Cleland JG. Clinical events leading to the progression of heart failure: insights from a national database of hospital discharges. *Eur Heart J*. 2001;22:153–164.

14. Howell MD, Geraci JM, Knowlton AA. Congestive heart failure and outpatient risk of venous thromboembolism: a retrospective, case-control study. *J Clin Epidemiol*. 2001;54:810–816.

15. Teerlink JR. Dyspnea as an end point in clinical trials of therapies for acute decompensated heart failure [review]. *Am Heart J*. 2003;145(Suppl 2):S26–S33.

16. Rostagno C, Olivo G, Comeglio M, et al. Prognostic value of 6-minute walk corridor test in patients with mild to moderate heart failure: comparison with other methods of functional evaluation. *Eur J Heart Fail*. 2003;5:247–252.

17. Forman DE, Butler J, Wang Y, et al. Incidence, predictors at admission, and impact of worsening renal function among patients hospitalized with heart failure. *J Am Coll Cardiol*. 2004;43:61–67.

18. Marantz PR, Kaplan MC, Alderman MH. Clinical diagnosis of congestive heart failure in patients with acute dyspnea. *Chest*. 1990;97:776–781.

19. Peacock WF IV, Albert NM, Kies P, White RD, Emerman CL. Bioimpedance monitoring: better than chest x-ray for predicting abnormal pulmonary fluid? *Congest Heart Fail*. 2000;6:86–89.

20. Kearney MT, Zaman A, Eckberg DL, et al. Cardiac size, autonomic function, and 5-year follow-up of chronic heart failure patients with severe prolongation of ventricular activation. *J Card Fail.* 2003;9:93–99.

21. Cheng V, Kazanagra R, Garcia A, et al. A rapid bedside test for B-type peptide predicts treatment outcomes in patients admitted for decompensated heart failure: a pilot study. *J Am Coll Cardiol.* 2001;37:386–391.

22. Potluri S, Ventura HO, Mulumudi M, Mehra MR. Cardiac troponin levels in heart failure. *Cardiol Rev.* 2004;12:21–25.

23. Lee DS, Austin PC, Rouleau JL, et al. Predicting mortality among patients hospitalized for heart failure: derivation and validation of a clinical model. *JAMA.* 2003;290: 2581–2587.

Heart Failure Discharge Declaration

Patient Name: _____

Attending Physician: _____

I understand that there are several steps I can take to help keep myself healthy and prevent another heart failure hospitalization. These steps include:

Taking My Medications

After I leave the hospital, I will continue to take my medications.

I also will report any reactions (side effects) I think are caused by my medications to:

_____ at _____
(name)   (contact information)

☐ I have been given a list of the current medications that I am to take.

Taking Care of Myself

I also will follow the instructions given to me concerning:

☐ Diet
My doctor has recommended that I eat a _____ gram sodium diet with the following specifics:
_____

☐ Fluid Restriction
My doctor has recommended that I restrict my fluid intake to _____ each 24 hours.

☐ Daily Weights
My doctor has recommended that I have a scale at home and measure and record my weight at approximately the same time each day.

☐ Physical Activity
My doctor has recommended that I exercise for _____ a day, _____ times a week.
A good exercise for me is: _____

☐ Smoking Cessation
My doctor has advised that I absolutely, positively not smoke cigarettes again.
To help me stop smoking, my doctor has suggested/prescribed: _____

☐ Scheduling Visits to My Doctor
Primary Care Doctor's name _____ Phone number _____
Cardiology Doctor's name _____ Phone number _____

My first visit should be scheduled: _____

I know that following my doctor's advice will help me live a longer, higher-quality, and healthier life.

Patient Signature: _____	Date: _____
Discharge Physician or Nurse Signature: _____	Date: _____

This sample template form is provided only as an example. You are solely responsible for determining the appropriateness of its use and the content of any form that you develop from it.

Adapted by The ADHERE Registry Scientific Advisory Committee and based on UCLA Medical Center's Patient Discharge Declaration.

Adhere

Patient Discharge Declaration

Page available in full form on CD

NURSING DISCHARGE SUMMARY:

Date: _____ Departure Time: _____

VS: BP_____ P_____ R_____ T_____(If abnormal, document intervention)

Last void: _____ am / pm   ☐NA

Discharged To: ☐ Home   ☐ Other_____

Mode of Transportation: From Unit: ☐ Ambulatory ☐ Wheelchair   ☐Other_____

From Hospital: ☐ Car   ☐Ambulance Other_____

Person Accompanying Patient:

   ☐Family Member-Relationship_____

   ☐Other_____

Escorted to Hospital Exit: ☐CMS   ☐Other_____

Discharge Instruction Form Given: ☐Yes   ☐NA

CPC Form (Home or ECF Completed: ☐Yes   ☐NA

Belongings Sent with Patient: ☐Family Member   ☐NA

   If No, Action Taken:_____

Prescriptions Given to: _____   ☐NA

ACP Evaluation Summary: ☐Yes   ☐No

Comments:

_____

_____

_____

_____

_____

_____

_____

_____

_____

_____

_____

_____

_____

_____

_____

_____

_____

_____

Page available in full form on CD

DISCHARGE INSTRUCTIONS
Observation Heart Failure

BOTSFORD GENERAL HOSPITAL
28050 Grand River Avenue
Farmington Hills, MI 48336-5933

Bring this form to your next doctor's appointment.

To treat and control your heart failure, your doctor has recommended that you follow the instructions listed below:

I.   ACTIVITIES OF DAILY LIVING:

A. **Weigh** yourself every morning. Call your doctor if you gain more than 2-3 lbs in one week.

B. **Balance rest & activity:** Continue to do the activities that you enjoy. Both activity and rest are important to the health of your heart. Balancing them is the key to reducing heart failure symptom.

C. Too much **sodium** will cause your body to retain fluid. Maintain a low sodium diet. Your sodium limit per day is 2 gm/day or _____.
Other diet restrictions: _____

D. Your ejection fraction (heart function) : _____ ___%.

E. You are instructed to follow-up with your physician regarding the **pneumonia vaccine**.

F. **Smoking** increases your chances of developing illnesses that can shorten your life. You have been instructed to stop smoking.

G. **Driving:** ☐No restrictions
☐Special instructions: _____
_____

H. **Return to work:** ☐Not applicable
☐Special Instructions: _____

II.   DISCHARGE MEDICATIONS: Prescriptions given to: ☐Patient ☐Other _____
Take the following medications:

Name of Medication	Dose	Frequency

III.   FOLLOW-UP APPOINTMENT:
☐Return to your family doctor in _____ weeks. ☐Return to Cardiologist _____ in 48 hours.
Phone # _____
"Special Instructions" _____
Educational Material Provided: _____
☐Cardiac Rehab: You have been recommended to enroll in Cardiac Rehab. Please call for an appointment. Phone #: (248) 471-8342.
• If you experience :
  • Increase in shortness of breath
  • Increase in swelling in your legs or abdomen
  • Have a cough that does not go away and gets worse when you lie down
  • Chest Pain, palpitation or dizziness
GO TO THE NEAREST EMERGENCY ROOM

_____   _____
Physician Signature   Date/Time   RN Signature   Date/Time
I have read and understand the above instructions. If I am unable to follow these instructions or have any questions I will call my doctor. I understand that these instructions are not all inclusive. _____
_____
Patient/Family Signature   Date

White – Chart   Yellow – patient's copy   Pink - physician

Obs. Heart Failure-Discharge Inst/h/dm/Discharge Inst/6/24/2005

Page available in full form on CD

Botsford General Hospital
CONGESTIVE HEART FAILURE
Discharge Teaching Instructions

If you have been diagnosed with heart failure, it's important to follow your doctor's advice exactly. Following your treatment plan can help you feel better, stay out of the hospital, and live longer.

Topic	Instructions
☒ Activity	• Remain physically active following your doctor's instructions about exercise and activity. • Rest often. Any time you become even a little tired or short of breath, SIT DOWN and rest. • Plan your activities to include rest periods. • Take note of your breathing pattern and how well you tolerate activity.
☒ Diet/Nutrition	• Limit your salt intake. Too much salt will cause swelling and could make it harder for you to breathe. Use salt substitutes ONLY if your doctor permits. • Follow any diet instructions given to you by your doctor or the dietitian including how much salt (sodium) you are allowed each day. • If you are overweight, talk to your doctor about a weight reduction plan. • You may need to limit how much fluid you drink. Remember: things that melt like ice cream, Jell-O or ice, still count as fluids!
☒ Medications	• Your doctor may prescribe one or a combination of medications for you. • You MUST take medicine every day to treat congestive heart failure. Be sure to take your **medicines exactly as your doctor tells you: no more, no less.** • Skipping doses or not refilling a prescription could cause serious problems. Do not stop taking your medicine without talking to your doctor. • Medicines sometimes cause side effects like causing you to cough or go to the bathroom more often. If you have side effects or questions or believe the medicine is not helping you call your doctor.
☒ Follow-up	Be sure and schedule a follow-up appointment with your primary care doctor or any specialists as instructed.
☒ Weight Monitoring	• Weigh yourself every day at the same time with the same amount of clothing on. • If you notice a consistent weight gain (2 lbs. In 2 days), call your doctor at once.
Call your doctor if:	• **Alert your doctor any time you notice a change in your body or your symptoms**, but be especially aware of the following and call your doctor if any of these signs or symptoms occur or if you experience any other new symptoms: ✓ Trouble breathing, especially during activity or when lying flat In bed ✓ Waking up out of breath at night ✓ Frequent dry, hacking cough, especially when lying down ✓ Feeling tired, weak, faint or dizzy ✓ Swollen feet, ankles and legs ✓ Nausea, with stomach swelling, pain and tenderness • **If you experience chest pain, go to the nearest emergency room immediately.**
☒ Smoking	• **Do not smoke or use other tobacco products.** Tobacco is probably the single most dangerous thing you can do to your health. Nicotine robs the heart of oxygen and constricts blood vessels, which raises heart rate and blood pressure. If you smoke or use tobacco products, discuss alternatives with your doctor. The most important thing is that you continue to try to quit until you are successful! • **Michigan Tobacco Quit Line** – 1-800-480-QUIT (7848)
☒ Additional Instructions	• Avoid people with colds and flu. • Keep all appointments. • Work with your doctor. To get the most benefit from your health care, you need to take an active role. Visit your doctor regularly, take notes, and ask questions.

I have reviewed the above information with my nurse. My questions regarding this information have been answered to my satisfaction. My signature on this form indicates that I have received and understand the above information.

_____   _____

Patient Signature   Date   Discharging Nurse's Signature   Date
Or Responsible Person if Patient Unable to Sign

Congestive Heart Failure Discharge Teaching Inst/h/dm/Discharge Inst/6/15/2005

Page available in full form on CD

Putting It All Together: Guidelines to Life with Heart Failure

No matter how severe your heart failure is, there are many things you can do to control the condition. You will enjoy a better quality of life when you follow your doctors' recommendations for your medications, diet and exercise.

Medication

- ♥ Take your medications as prescribed by your doctor. If you miss a dose, don't take two the next time.
- ♥ Always review over-the-counter medications with your doctor, nurse or pharmacist before taking them.

Diet

Eating too much salt and drinking alcohol are the most common cause for hospitalizations in people with heart failure.

- ♥ Follow your prescribed diet. For most patients, this means limiting sodium to 2,000 milligrams (2 grams) each day.
- ♥ See a registered dietitian if you have problems with, or questions about, your diet.
- ♥ Avoid alcohol, it is harmful for people with heart failure.

Weight

- ♥ Weigh yourself every day in the morning, before eating, after going to the bathroom.
- ♥ Write your weight down in your "diary".
- ♥ Call your doctor if you gain or lose more than 2 to 3 pounds in one week.

Exercise

- ♥ Balance rest and exercise.
- ♥ formal exercise in your daily routine.
- ♥ Heart failure gets worse in people who stop exercising.

Vaccinations

- ♥ Get a flu shot each year (October or November are the best times).
- ♥ Talk to your doctor about a shot to prevent pneumonia ("pneumovax").

Smoking

If you smoke, one of the best things you can do for your health is to stop smoking. Smoking is hard on your heart because it reduces the amount of oxygen in your blood, damages your blood vessels and causes your heart to beat too fast.

- ♥ Ask your doctor about programs to help you quit smoking.
- ♥ Find sources of support and encouragement such as friends, family, support groups or smoking cessation programs.
- ♥ Don't use smokeless tobacco (snuff or chew); they can be as harmful to your health as smoking.

Heart Failure Warning Signs

- ▸ If you experience any of these, your heart failure may be getting worse. **Call your doctor or nurse if you...**
- ▸ gain or lose more than 2 to 3 pounds in one week
- ▸ have an increase in shortness of breath
- ▸ have an increase in swelling in your legs or abdomen
- ▸ have a cough that does not go away or gets worse when you lie down
- ▸ have any side effects from your medications
- ▸ have any sense of feeling worse

Call your doctor or nurse any time you have questions or concerns. Most problems can be easily treated either over the phone or with a visit to the doctor's office. Don't let warning signs go untreated. Bad things usually just get worse if they go unattended, and you could end up being admitted to hospital unnecessarily.

Long-term Outlook

It is impossible to determine the long-term outlook for an individual. Prognosis, or long-term outlook, is based on many factors, including:

- ♥ the cause of heart failure
- ♥ the severity of heart failure
- ♥ the duration of heart failure
- ♥ the response to treatment

Although there are no easy answers, it is possible to control heart failure and improve your quality of life.

Page available in full form on CD

To Our Valued Patient,

It has been the custom of Botsford General Hospital to reach out to the people of the community and provide programs to meet their needs. As part of our heart Failure Program, Botsford Hospital offers a variety of programs and classes to enrich your health care needs. You may wish to discuss these programs with your physician to decide which services are right for you.

❖ **The Breather's Club**

Purpose: To provide information and support to anyone with lung disease.

When: The 3rd Thursday of every month at 1:00pm

Where: Conference room 2 East

Cost: There is no fee

For more information, call (XXX)XXX-XXXX

❖ **Cardiac Rehabilitation**

Purpose: To provide a series of phased activities designed to help patients and their families gain health benefits by managing their diet, exercise and attitudes toward heart conditions.

Where: Classes are held on 2 West

Cost: The cost varies, depending on your insurance coverage.

For more information, call (XXX)XXX-XXXX

❖ **Pulmonary Rehabilitation**

Purpose: To provide education, support and to increase activity, endurance and tolerance for patients with pulmonary disease.

Where: Classes are held on 2 West

Cost: The cost varies, depending on your insurance coverage.

For more information, call (XXX)XXX-XXXX

❖ <u>Health and Lifestyle Classes at health Development Network</u>

Purpose: To provide education programs for patients, families and the community in areas of health promotion, wellness and disease management. HDN's staff are health professionals such as nurses, dieticians, social workers.

Note: You may receive a letter from this department after you leave the hospital if your doctor or nurse has referred you to a program.

When: Classes and individual consultations are scheduled at a variety of times convenient for most individuals. Day, evening and Saturday appointments are available.

Cost: Fees vary depending on the type of program. HDN staff will work to help if there is difficulty with program fees.

Programs offered include: Stop Smoking, Stress Management, Nutrition programs and consultation including low sodium and weight management, Healthy Cooking demonstrations, Diabetes Management, Blood Pressure and Cholesterol Screening, Breather's Education. Quarterly Community calendars list programs, dates and times.

For more information, call (XXX)XXX-XXXX

Patient Reminder Card

For best results, please print on heavyweight paper. Cut along black dotted lines and roll fold at blue dotted lines for a 4-paneled, 3-fold 2" x 3.5" pocket card. To receive additional pocket cards, please call 1-866-616-2993.

FRONT

Patient Reminder Card

Patient Name

BACK

ADHERE is a registered trademark of Scios Inc. and pending before the USPTO.
©2004 Scios Inc. All rights reserved.

Appointments

DATE — TIME

REMINDER
Always maintain a low-salt diet.

- Increase in shortness of breath
- Swelling in the legs or ankles
- Weight gain ≥3 lbs within a few days
- Difficulty breathing when lying down
- Worsening tiredness
- Stomach bloating/fullness and loss of appetite
- Dry cough, especially when lying down

Adhere
Acute Decompensated Heart Failure National Registry

CALL

Dr. _____
at (___) _____

if you have signs or symptoms of worsening CHF

Medications

MEDICATIONS	STRENGTH	DOSING

From The ADHERE®
Scientific Advisory Committee

Medications

MEDICATION	STRENGTH	DOSING

Page available in full form on CD

Pocket Cards
RAPID Heart Failure Assessment Guide

For best results, please print on heavyweight paper. Cut along black dotted lines and roll fold at blue dotted lines for a 6" x 4" card. To receive additional pocket cards, please call 1-866-616-2993.

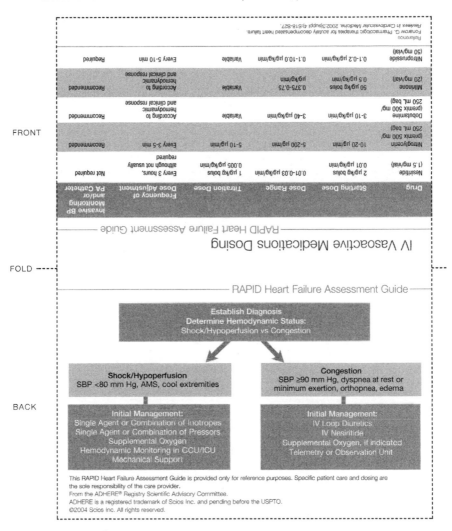

Page available in full form on CD

Pocket Cards
IV Vasoactive Medications Pocket Card

For best results, please print on heavyweight paper. Cut along black dotted lines and roll fold at blue dotted lines for a 6" x 4" card. To receive additional pocket cards, please call 1-866-616-2993.

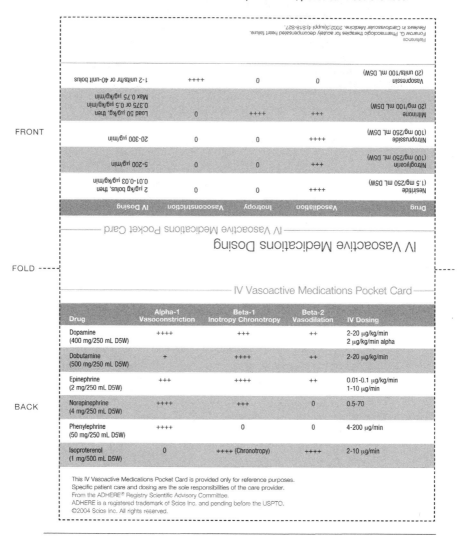

FRONT

Reference
Forsarow G. Pharmacologic therapies for acutely decompensated heart failure. *Reviews in Cardiovascular Medicine.* 2002;3(suppl 4):S18-S27.

Drug	Vasodilation	Inotropy	Vasoconstriction	IV Dosing
Nesiritide (1.5 mg/250 mL D5W)	++++	0	0	2 µg/kg bolus, then 0.01-0.03 µg/kg/min
Nitroglycerin (100 mg/250 mL D5W)	+++	0	0	5-200 µg/min
Nitroprusside (100 mg/250 mL D5W)	++++	0	0	20-300 µg/min
Milrinone (20 mg/100 mL D5W)	+++	++++	0	Load 50 µg/kg, then 0.375 or 0.5 µg/kg/min Max 0.75 µg/kg/min
Vasopressin (20 units/100 mL D5W)	0	0	++++	1-2 units/hr or 40-unit bolus

IV Vasoactive Medications Dosing
—— IV Vasoactive Medications Pocket Card ——

FOLD

—— IV Vasoactive Medications Pocket Card ——

BACK

Drug	Alpha-1 Vasoconstriction	Beta-1 Inotropy Chronotropy	Beta-2 Vasodilation	IV Dosing
Dopamine (400 mg/250 mL D5W)	++++	+++	++	2-20 µg/kg/min 2 µg/kg/min alpha
Dobutamine (500 mg/250 mL D5W)	+	++++	++	2-20 µg/kg/min
Epinephrine (2 mg/250 mL D5W)	+++	++++	++	0.01-0.1 µg/kg/min 1-10 µg/min
Norepinephrine (4 mg/250 mL D5W)	++++	+++	0	0.5-70
Phenylephrine (50 mg/250 mL D5W)	++++	0	0	4-200 µg/min
Isoproterenol (1 mg/500 mL D5W)	0	++++ (Chronotropy)	++++	2-10 µg/min

This IV Vasoactive Medications Pocket Card is provided only for reference purposes.
Specific patient care and dosing are the sole responsibilities of the care provider.
From the ADHERE® Registry Scientific Advisory Committee.
ADHERE is a registered trademark of Scios Inc. and pending before the USPTO.
©2004 Scios Inc. All rights reserved.

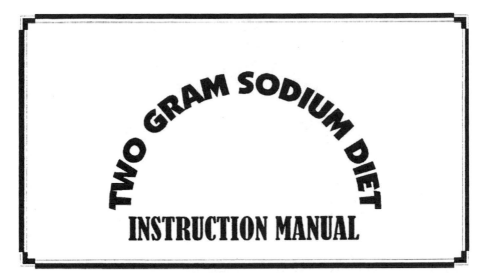

TWO GRAM SODIUM DIET
INSTRUCTION MANUAL

PATIENT'S NAME:_____   **DIETITIAN'S NAME:**_____

DIETITIAN'S PHONE NUMBER:_____

THIS BROCHURE PRODUCED BY
THE CLINICAL NUTRITION SERVICES DEPARTMENT AT
BOTSFORD GENERAL HOSPITAL

Page available in full form on CD

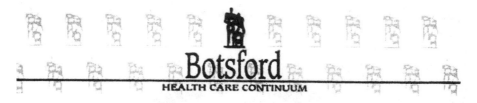

COMMON QUESTIONS ASKED ABOUT THE
2 GRAM SODIUM DIET

1. WHAT IS SODIUM?
This is an essential mineral to the body. It helps the body regulate fluid balance.

2. WHY IS IT IMPORTANT THAT I REDUCE MY SODIUM INTAKE?
Under certain conditions, such as heart disease, high blood pressure, and renal disease, the intake of excess sodium can cause the body to retain too much fluid. Every time you eat extra sodium, water is drawn out of the body's tissues to dilute it, causing more fluid buildup. In summary, living with these conditions is MUCH easier when you follow these sodium guidelines.

3. WHAT HAPPENS WHEN THERE IS FLUID BUILDUP IN MY BODY?
This means you experience more swelling (edema), and an increase in shortness of breath. And with more fluid, it is more difficult for the body to absorb your medications, so therefore your medicine becomes less effective.

4. WHERE IS SODIUM FOUND?
Sodium is found naturally in every food we eat. However, most of the sodium in our diet is added, usually as table salt. It is also found in many baking ingredients and medications. This information will provide you with guidelines to reducing your overall sodium intake.

Page available in full form on CD

botsford
general
hospital

YOUR GUIDE TO
THE NEW FOOD LABEL

The new food label will carry an up-to-date, easier-to-use nutrition information guide, to be required on almost all packaged foods (compared to about 60 percent of products until now). The guide will serve as a key to help in planning a healthy diet.

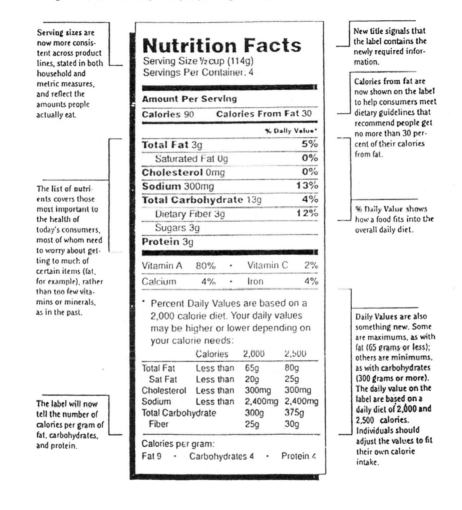

Serving sizes are now more consistent across product lines, stated in both household and metric measures, and reflect the amounts people actually eat.

The list of nutrients covers those most important to the health of today's consumers, most of whom need to worry about getting to much of certain items (fat, for example), rather than too few vitamins or minerals, as in the past.

The label will now tell the number of calories per gram of fat, carbohydrates, and protein.

New title signals that the label contains the newly required information.

Calories from fat are now shown on the label to help consumers meet dietary guidelines that recommend people get no more than 30 percent of their calories from fat.

% Daily Value shows how a food fits into the overall daily diet.

Daily Values are also something new. Some are maximums, as with fat (65 grams or less); others are minimums, as with carbohydrates (300 grams or more). The daily value on the label are based on a daily diet of 2,000 and 2,500 calories. Individuals should adjust the values to fit their own calorie intake.

Nutrition Facts

Serving Size ½ cup (114g)
Servings Per Container. 4

Amount Per Serving

Calories 90	Calories From Fat 30

	% Daily Value*
Total Fat 3g	5%
Saturated Fat 0g	0%
Cholesterol 0mg	0%
Sodium 300mg	13%
Total Carbohydrate 13g	4%
Dietary Fiber 3g	12%
Sugars 3g	
Protein 3g	

Vitamin A	80%	•	Vitamin C	2%
Calcium	4%	•	Iron	4%

* Percent Daily Values are based on a 2,000 calorie diet. Your daily values may be higher or lower depending on your calorie needs:

	Calories	2,000	2,500
Total Fat	Less than	65g	80g
Sat Fat	Less than	20g	25g
Cholesterol	Less than	300mg	300mg
Sodium	Less than	2,400mg	2,400mg
Total Carbohydrate		300g	375g
Fiber		25g	30g

Calories per gram:
Fat 9 • Carbohydrates 4 • Protein 4

Page available in full form on CD

WHAT ARE THE BASIC GUIDELINES FOR THIS DIET?

1. **DO NOT** USE TABLE SALT!
   Table salt is 40% sodium. JUST ONE TEASPOON contains 2300mg (2.3 grams) of sodium. This is more than the sodium level prescribed by your physician.

2. **DO NOT** ADD SALT IN COOKING! *(THIS CAN BE ELIMINATED FROM ANY RECIPE EXCEPT ONE CONTAINING YEAST)*

3. **DO** READ FOOD LABELS TO MONITOR YOUR SODIUM INTAKE.

4. **LIMIT** THE USE OF COMMERCIALLY PREPARED CONDIMENTS OR SALAD DRESSINGS, UNLESS THE PRODUCT STATES "NO SALT ADDED.
   (or 1 serving contains less than 200 mg)

5. **DO** PURCHASE A LOW SODIUM COOKBOOK TO PROVIDE GUIDELINES TO COOKING MEALS LOW SODIUM AND PALATABLE

6. **DO** MAKE USE OF HERBS AND SPICES INSTEAD OF SALT

7. **DO** FOLLOW THE "DINING OUT" GUIDELINES INCLUDED IN THIS BOOKLET.

8. **DO** KEEP THIS BOOK NEAR YOUR KITCHEN AS A GUIDE AND A REMINDER!

9. **WEIGH YOURSELF OFTEN, AS SUGGESTED BY YOUR DOCTOR TO MONITOR FOR EXCESS FLUID GAINS!!**

10. **CALL YOU DIETITIAN SHOULD _ANY_ QUESTIONS ARISE REGARDING YOUR DIET AS PRESCRIBED. A DIETITIAN CAN BE REACHED BY CALLING 248-471-8221.**

Page available in full form on CD

GENERAL GUIDELINES TO LABEL READING

1. Legal Definitions for the following terms:

Sodium Free – less than 5 mg per standard serving, can't contain any sodium chloride
(also known as table salt)
Very Low Sodium – 35mg or less sodium per standard serving
Low Sodium – 140 mg or less per standard serving
Reduced Sodium – At least 25% less sodium than in regular food
Light in Sodium – 50% less sodium per standard serving than in regular food
Unsalted or No Salt Added – No salt added in the processing, STILL has sodium
AND it may contain a substantial amount
Lightly Salted – 50% less added sodium than is normally added. This product
Will state NOT a low sodium food if that criteria is not met.

2. Nutrition Label

This will state the sodium content of foods, in milligrams (mg) per serving

3. Suggestions To Reading The Food Label

1. Look at the number of servings in the given package
   (i.e. – If you were reading the back of a soup can, it would state how many servings are in that can under the heading "serving")
2. Now you want to determine how much of that product you will eat
3. You then want to look at how much sodium is in EACH serving
4. REMEMBER that the label ONLY records the amount PER SERVING.
5. If you are going to consume the entire package and there are three servings, you will need to multiply the milligrams of sodium stated times three
   (i.e.- If the label states there is 100mg of sodium in one serving, and there are three servings in the box, and you wish to eat the entire box, you will want to take 100mg and multiply this times 3. This will let you know that there is 300mg of sodium in the box)

4. To Choose Appropriate Foods, You Will Want To Look For Foods That Contain 200mg Sodium or Less Per Serving

If you are consciously reading labels aim for no more than 700mg of sodium per meal

HERE IS A LIST OF LOW SODIUM COOKBOOKS YOU MAY FIND WORTHWHILE TO PURCHASE

AMERICAN HEART ASSOCIATION LOW SALT COOKBOOK: A COMPLETE GUIDE TO REDUCING SODIUM AND FAT Author- Rodman D. Starke (CURRENT RETAIL PRICE = $5.99)

INDIAN RECIPES FOR A HEALTHY HEART:140 LOW FAT, LOW SALT, LOW CHOLESTEROL GOURMET INDIAN DISHES Author- Mrs. Lakhani (CURRENT RETAIL PRICE = $11.96)

SECRETS TO LOW SALT COOKING Author – Jeanne Jones (CURRENT RETAIL PRICE =$11.95)

DELICIOUSLY SIMPLE: Quick and Easy low-sodium, low-fat, low cholesterol, low-sugar meals Author– Harriet Roth (CURRENT RETAIL PRICE = $11.95)

HARRIET ROTH'S DELICIOUSLY HEALTHY JEWISH COOKING: 350 Recipes Author- Harriet Roth (CURRENT RETAIL PRICE = $16.95)

MICROWAVE CUISINE COOKS LOW SODIUM Author – Millie Delahunty (CURRENT RETAIL PRICE = 2.95)

HEALTHY SNACKS:low-fat, low-sodium, low-sugar (CURRENT RETAIL PRICE = $6.95)

*This list was compiled 9/98. This is just a sampling of what is available. For more info, contact the clinical nutrition services department at Botsford General Hospital

** VISIT YOUR LOCAL LIBRARY OR BOOKSTORE FOR A MORE EXTENSIVE LIST

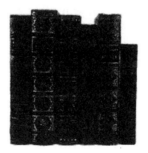

CHOOSING FOODS FOR A REDUCED SODIUM DIET

	CHOOSE	AVOID
BREADS (1 SERVING = 1 SLICE OF BREAD)	English muffin, white, wheat, pumpernickel, other types of regular or unsalted bread and rolls, unseasoned bread crumbs *(1 SERVING CONTAINS APPROX. 100-150 MG SODIUM)*	Sweet rolls, breads or rolls with salted tops, packaged cracker or bread crumb coatings, packaged stuffing mixes, biscuits, corn bread *(1 SERVING CONTAINS APPROX. 200-300MG SODIUM)*
CEREALS (1 SERVING = ½ CUP)	**Regular cooked cereals, such as** oats, cream of wheat, rice **Cold cereals, such as** shredded wheat, puffed wheat, puffed rice, low sodium corn flakes and rice krispies *(1 SERVING CONTAINS APPROX. 0-150 MG SODIUM)*	**INSTANT** hot cereals, any other ready-to-eat cereals (important to read label) *(1 SERVING CONTAINS APPROX. 280-400MG SODIUM)*
CRACKERS/ SNACK FOODS (1 SERVING = 1 OUNCE SNACK FOODS)	**ALL** unsalted crackers & snack foods, unsalted peanut butter *(1 SERVING CONTAINS APPROX. 35 MG SODIUM)*	Salted crackers, Potato chips, salted pretzels, ready made party dips and spreads *(1 SERVING CONTAINS APPROX. 300+ MG SODIUM PER SERVING)*
PASTA, RICE, & POTATOES (1 SERVING = 1 CUP)	**ALL** types of pastas (macaroni, spaghetti, ziti, etc…), plain potatoes, plain rice *(1 SERVING CONTAINS APPROX. 1 MG SODIUM)*	Macaroni and cheese mix; seasoned rice mix; noodle and spaghetti mixes; canned spaghetti; frozen lasagna, instant potatoes, instant pasta salad mixes *(1 SERVING CONTAINS APPROX. 800-1000 MG SODIUM)*
DRIED BEANS &PEAS (1 SERVING = 1 CUP COOKED)	Pinto beans, white northern beans, split peas, etc… *(1 SERVING CONTAINS APPROX. 15 MG SODIUM)*	Any beans prepared with **ham, bacon, salt pork, or bacon grease. All canned beans** *(1 SERVING CONTAINS APPROX. 800 – 1200 MG SODIUM)*

Page available in full form on CD

CHOOSING FOODS FOR A REDUCED SODIUM DIET (CONT'D)

	CHOOSE	AVOID
MEATS/ MEAT ALTERNATIVES (1 SERVING = 3 OUNCE PORTION SIZE)	Fresh or frozen meat, poultry and fish; Low sodium canned tuna and salmon; eggs *(1 SERVING CONTAINS APPROX. 60-50 MG SODIUM)*	**Salted, smoked, canned, spiced, and pickled meats, poultry and fish** **Ham, bacon, sausage** **Regular canned tuna or salmon** **Cold cuts, luncheon meats; hot dogs; pre-breaded frozen meats, fish, poultry; TV dinners; meat pies; kosher meats**
FRUITS AND VEGETABLES (1 SERVING = 1 CUP COOKED VEGETABLES, ½ CUP JUICE, 1 MEDIUM SIZE PIECE FRUIT)	Fresh, frozen, or low-sodium canned vegetables or vegetable juices; low sodium tomato paste and sauce; fresh, canned, or frozen fruit and juices *(1 SERVING CONTAINS APPROX. 1-20 MG SODIUM)*	**Regular canned** vegetables, regular tomato juice and tomato paste, olives, pickles, sauerkraut, or vegetables packed in **brine** Frozen vegetables in **butter and sauces** **Crystallized or glazed** fruit, maraschino cherries, fruit dried with **SODIUM SULFITE**
DAIRY PRODUCTS (1 SERVING = 8 OUNCE MILK, 8 OUNCE YOGURT, 1 OUNCE CHEESE)	Milk, cream, sour cream, non-dairy creamer, yogurt, low sodium cottage cheese, low sodium cheese *(I SERVING CONTAINS APPROX. 150 MG PER SERVING)* **Limit** margarine, regular butter or mayonnaise to **4 teaspoons per day!**	Buttermilk, dutch processed chocolate milk, processed cheese slices and spreads, regular cheese, regular cottage cheese
FATS AND OILS (1 SERVING = 1 TBSP)	Unsalted butter, unsalted margarine, cooking oils, or shortenings; salt free gravies, low sodium salad dressing	Bacon grease; salt pork; commercially prepared sauces, gravies, and salad dressings

Page available in full form on CD

CHOOSING FOODS FOR A REDUCED SODIUM DIET (CONT'D)

	CHOOSE	AVOID
BEVERAGES	Coffee, tea, fruit flavored drinks **NOT** containing sodium	Softened water, carbonated beverages that are not noted as low sodium
SOUPS	Salt-free soups, low sodium bouillon cubes	Regular commercially canned or prepared soups, stews, broths, and bouillon; packaged and frozen soups
DESSERTS	Gelatin, sherbert, fruit ices, pudding, angel food cake, salt-free baked goods, sugar, jelly, syrup, ice cream	Regular commercially prepared and packaged baked goods; chocolate candy
CONDIMENTS	Fresh and dried herbs Lemon juice Low-sodium mustard, vinegar, low-sodium, or no salt added ketchup; seasoning blends that do not contain salt	**Table salt, lite salt. Bouillon cubes, meat extract, Worcestershire sauce, tarter sauce, ketchup, chili sauce, cooking wines, onion salt, prepared mustard, garlic salt, meat flavorings, meat tenderizers, steak and barbecue sauce, seasoned salt, MSG, Dutch processed cocoa**

Page available in full form on CD

SODIUM CONTENT IN COMMON FOODS
***FOODS WITH 0-200 MG SODIUM PER SERVING *ARE ACCEPTABLE* ***FOODS WITH MORE THAN 200 MG PER SERVING *ARE NOT ACCEPTABLE*

SEASONINGS	SODIUM CONTENT
1 TSP GARLIC POWDER	(1 MG SODIUM)
1 TBSP HORSERADISH, PREPARED	(165 MG SODIUM)
1 TSP GARLIC SALT	(2050 MG SODIUM)
1 TSP SALT	(2132 MG SODIUM)

CONDIMENTS	
1 TSP MUSTARD	(65 MG SODIUM)
1 TBSP LOW SODIUM KETCHUP	(90 MG SODIUM)
1 TSP BARBECUE SAUCE	(127 MG SODIUM)
1 TBSP. KETCHUP	(178 MG SODIUM)
1 TBSP LITE SOY SAUCE	(600 MG SODIUM)
1 TBSP REGULAR SOY SAOUCE	(1029 MG SODIUM)

CHEESE	
1 OUNCE CREAM CHEESE	(85 MG SODIUM)
1 OUNCE BRICK CHEESE	(159 MG SODIUM)
1 OUNCE MUENSTER CHEESE	(178 MG SODIUM)
1 CUP RICOTTA CHEESE	(208 MG SODIUM)
1 OUNCE BLUE CHEESE	(394 MG SODIUM)
1 OUNCE ROQUEFORT CHEESE	(512 MG SODIUM)
1 CUP COTTAGE CHEESE	(918 MG SODIUM)

BEVERAGES	
REGULAR SODA	(10 MG SODIUM)
DIET SODA	(30 MG SODIUM)
MILK, 8 OUNCES	(120 MG SODIUM)
COCOA MIX	(201 MG SODIUM)
BUTTERMILK	(257 MG SODIUM)

MEATS	
FISH, BAKED, 3 OUNCES	(54 MG SODIUM)
BEEF, 3 OUNCES	(55 MG SODIUM)
EGGS	(63 MG SODIUM)
CHICKEN, ½ BREAST	(69 MG SODIUM)
SHRIMP, 3 OUNCES, RAW	(126 MG SODIUM)
FRIED FISH, 3 OUNCES	(238 MG SODIUM)
CORNED BEEF, 3 OUNCES	(972 MG SODIUM)

The arrows to the left of each section are labeled "LOW TO HIGH".

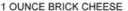

Page available in full form on CD

BREADS

HOT CEREAL (REGULAR)	(0 MG SODIUM)
KIX	(113 MG SODIUM)
LIFE CEREAL	(115 MG SODIUM)
1 SLICE BREAD	(120 MG SODIUM)
CHEERIOS, ½ CUP	(123 MG SODIUM)
1 BISCUIT	(308 MG SODIUM)
HOT CEREAL, INSTANT	(400+ MG SODIUM)
ALL BRAN	(481 MG SODIUM)

EXAMPLES OF SODIUM IN FAST FOODS

ARBY'S

FRENCH FRIES, SMALL	(114 MG SODIUM)
ROAST BEEF SANDWICH, REGULAR	(588 MG SODIUM)
SALAD, CHEF	(706 MG SODIUM)
LIGHT ROAST BEEF DELUXE	(826 MG SODIUM)
CHICKEN CORDON BLUE SANDWICH	(1824 MG SODIUM)

BURGER KING

SIDE SALAD	(27 MG SODIUM)
MINI MUFFINS , BLUEBERRY	(244 MG SODIUM
DIPPING SAUCE, BARBECUE	(397 MG SODIUM)
HAMBURGER, PLAIN	(505 MG SODIUM)
CHICKEN TENDERS	(641 MG SODIUM)
BK BROILER CHICKEN SANDWICH	(728 MG SODIUM)
WHOPPER WITH CHEESE	(1177 MG SODIUM)

KENTUCKY FRIED CHICKEN

CHICKEN LITTLES SANDWICH	(331 MG SODIUM)
BUTTERMILK BISCUIT	(655 MG SODIUM)
EXTRA CRISPY CENTER BREAST	(790 MG SODIUM)
KENTUCKY NUGGETS	(840 MG SODIUM)

McDONALD'S

FAT FREE APPLE MUFFIN	(200 MG SODIUM)
CHUNKY CHICKEN SALAD	(230 MG SODIUM)
CHICKEN FAJITAS	(310 MG SODIUM)
HAMBURGER	(490 MG SODIUM)

Page available in full form on CD

McDONALD'S (CONT'D)
EGG McMUFFIN   (710 MG SODIUM)
BIG MAC   (890 MG SODIUM)
QUARTER POUNDER WITH CHEESE (1090 MG SODIUM)

PIZZA HUT
2 SLICES THIN CHEESE PIZZA   (867 MG SODIUM)
2 SLICES PAN PIZZA, PEPPERONI   (1127 MG SODIUM)
2 SLICES PAN PIZZA, SUPREME   (1447 MG SODIUM
2 SLICES CHEESE PIZZA   (1276 MG SODIUM)

SUBWAY
SALAD, GARDEN, LARGE   (634 MG SODIUM)
SANDWICH, HAM, 6 INCH   (839 MG SODIUM)
SANDWICH, TURKEY, 6 INCH   (839 MG SODIUM)
SANDWICH, STEAK, 6 INCH   (1306 MG SODIUM)

TACO BELL
TACO, FIESTA, BEEF   (139 MG SODIUM)
TACO, SOFT CHICKEN   (615 MG SODIUM)
TACO SALAD, WITH SHELL   (910 MG SODIUM)
MEXICAN PIZZA   (1031 MG SODIUM)

WENDY'S
BAKED POTATO,   (135 MG SODIUM)
WITH SOUR CREAM & CHIVES
BAKED POTATO   (455 MG SODIUM)
WITH BROCCOLI & CHEESE
HAMBURGER, PLAIN   (500 MG SODIUM)
CHILI, 9 OZ   (750 MG SODIUM)
CHEESEBURGER   (760 MG SODIUM)
CHICKEN CLUB SANDWICH   (930 MG SODIUM)

***FOODS WITH 0-200 MG SODIUM PER SERVING <u>ARE ACCEPTABLE</u> IN YOUR DIET PLAN   ***FOODS WITH MORE THAN 200 MG PER SERVING ARE <u>NOT ACCEPTABLE</u>

Page available in full form on CD

SAMPLE MEAL PLAN FOR A 2 GRAM SODIUM DIET

10 STARCH SERVINGS PER DAY
3 FRUIT SERVINGS PER DAY
3 MILK SERVINGS PER DAY
2 VEGETABLE SERVINGS PER DAY
1 DESSERT PER DAY
6 MEAT SERVINGS PER DAY

***REMEMBER**, IF YOU ARE ON OTHER DIETARY RESTRICTIONS THIS SAMPLE **SHOULD NOT** BE FOLLOWED. YOU SHOULD CONTACT YOUR DIETITIAN FOR THE CORRECT MEAL PLAN.

BREAKFAST
¾ CUP CEREAL
1 SLICE WHOLE WHEAT TOAST
½ CUP ORANGE SECTIONS
2 tsp. UNSALTED MARGARINE
2 tsp. JELLY
1 CUP SKIM MILK
COFFEE
CREAMER/SUGAR

LUNCH
½ CUP CHICKEN NOODLE SOUP
3 OUNCE HAMBURGER
1 HAMBURGER BUN
2 OUNCES OF TOMATO SLICES
LETTUCE
1 tsp MAYONNAISE
3 UNSALTED CRACKERS
3 VANILLA WAFERS
½ CUP CANNED PEACHES
1 CUP SKIM MILK
COFFEE
CREAMER/SUGAR

DINNER
3 OUNCE BAKED CHICKEN BREAST
1 MEDIUM BAKED POTATO
½ CUP GREEN BEANS
TOSSED SALAD
1 Tbsp DIET ITALIAN DRESSING
1 SLICE WHOLE WHEAT BREAD
2 tsp UNSALTED MARGARINE
1 SLICE ANGEL FOOD CAKE
½ STRAWBERRIES

SNACK
1 UNSALTED SOFT PRETZEL
½ CUP APPLE JUICE

SAMPLE MENU PROVIDES:
CALORIES: 2170 KCAL
PROTEIN: 105 gm
CARBOHYDRATE: 300 gm
FAT: 55 gm
SODIUM: 1850 mg
POTASSIUM: 4450 mg

Page available in full form on CD

INDEX

Note: Pages followed by f indicate illustrations; those followed by t indicate tables.